Brown Sugar
and
Health

Also by Professor I. I. Brekhman

Man and Biologically Active Substances
The Effect of Drugs, Diet and Pollution on Health

The principal aim of this book is to show the role of biologically active substances (BAS) in people's health. Food and medicine constitute a multi-component BAS flow that establishes the most intimate relationship with the environment and builds up the inner ecology of the organism. Regulating the BAS flow is essential for the preservation of health.

In this book particular aspects are examined, such as the prophylaxis of morbidity, effective occupational activity, regulation of natality, and the preservation of health in hard and extreme conditions.

The book shows how wholesome food and the so-called 'medicines' for healthy people, are conflicting elements in man's fight to be healthy.

89 pages   198 literature references   ISBN 0 08 023169 1

Brown Sugar
and
Health

by

I. I. BREKHMAN and I. F. NESTERENKO

Department of Physiology and Pharmacology of Adaptation
Institute of Marine Biology, Far-East Scientific Centre
Academy of Sciences of the USSR, Vladivostock

Translator

J. H. APPLEBY

Translation Editor

J. HICKLIN

PERGAMON PRESS

OXFORD · NEW YORK · TORONTO · SYDNEY · PARIS · FRANKFURT

U.K.	Pergamon Press Ltd., Headington Hill Hall, Oxford OX3 0BW, England
U.S.A.	Pergamon Press Inc., Maxwell House, Fairview Park, Elmsford, New York 10523, U.S.A.
CANADA	Pergamon Press Canada Ltd., Suite 104, 150 Consumers Rd., Willowdale, Ontario M2J 1P9, Canada
AUSTRALIA	Pergamon Press (Aust.) Pty. Ltd., P.O. Box 544, Potts Point, N.S.W. 2011, Australia
FRANCE	Pergamon Press SARL, 24 rue des Ecoles, 75240 Paris, Cedex 05, France
FEDERAL REPUBLIC OF GERMANY	Pergamon Press GmbH, 6242 Kronberg-Taunus, Hammerweg 6, Federal Republic of Germany

Translation copyright © 1983 Pergamon Press Ltd.

First English edition 1983

Library of Congress Cataloging in Publication Data
Brekhman, I. I. (Izrail'Itsikovich), 1921-
Brown Sugar and Health.
At head of title: Department of Physiology and Pharmacology of Adaptation. Institute of Marine Biology. Far-East Scientific Centre. Academy of Sciences of the USSR, Vladivostock.
Includes bibliographical references and index.
1. Sugar. I. Nesterenko, I. F. II. Hicklin, J.
III. Title.
TX560.S9B73 1982   641.3'36   82-16674

British Library Cataloguing in Publication Data
Brekhman, I. I.
Brown Sugar and Health.
1. Sugar—Physiological effect
I. Title   II. Nesterenko, I. F.
613.2'6   TX560.S9
ISBN 0-08-026837-4

Printed in Great Britain by A. Wheaton & Co. Ltd., Exeter

Contents

Introduction

As it turns out I have spent all my 35 years as a pharmacologist study-ing medicines that are not 'high-flyers'. These substances, which are individual natural medicines as opposed to synthetic chemical com-posites, do not have immediate and spectacular effects: by contrast, their effects develop slowly. Moreover, because they are meant not so much for the sick as for the healthy they have not been able to pride themselves on the cure of any particular illnesses. These factors com-bined have posed formidable difficulties, for myself, my colleagues and all those who have followed in our footsteps. It has taken agoniz-ingly long, over 30 years of constant research fraught with problems, for the legendary value of ginseng to win recognition by scientists and doctors. Eleutherococcus, a more than worthy substitute for ginseng, won acclaim considerably faster, nevertheless we had to devote a quarter of a century of study to it. The story of rantarin (a medicinal substance like pantocrin extracted from the non-ossified antlers of the European reindeer) and the other medicines which my late teacher Professor N.V. Lazarev named adaptogens is no less long and eventful.

The greatest difficulties have arisen, however, from the fact that these substances are not synthesized in the laboratory; nor are they extracted from plants and animals as isolated substances: they are chemically complex, with a lot of components. There are many reasons why scientists and technicians have given preference to simple (pure) substances. They are the pride and joy of the chemists who synthesize them; pharmacologists find them easy to handle — there are no problems determining dosages and tissue concentrations, evaluating their pharmacokinetics is straightforward, and so on. Synthetic medi-cines store relatively well and are fairly easy to assess by quality and quantity. But as we pay our well deserved tribute to the many syn-thetic remedies that have rendered great service to mankind we should not overlook the circumstance that most of the positive aspects of synthetic medicines favour their producers not their consumers. What is more, the brain children of the modern pharmaceutical industry are responsible for many harmful effects — drug-induced disease and the spread of allergization, among others. Of course, when serious diseases require treatment and it is a matter of life and death, powerful and fast-acting drugs must be deployed, regardless of whether they are completely safe. But it is another matter when people are obliged to resort to medicines in everyday life, for, say, depression or anxiety, for preventing atherosclerosis or for controlling small deviations of arterial pressure. In addition, there are clearly occasions when healthy people need to take medicines, likewise those individuals who hover in a state somewhere between health and illness. It is also obvious that medicines represent only one form of the biologically active substances entering the body, most of which take the form of food.

These and other considerations have led to the notion that pharmacology as an applied science has two aspects. In the past pharmacotherapy, the pharmacology of illness, has been developed preferentially. However, leaving aside the last few decades, the pharmacology of health — health pharmacology, which I have named *pharmacosanation* — has no less venerable roots. It is probable that I came to appreciate the importance of this 'other pharmacology' precisely because the medicines that I happened to have investigated were chiefly meant for healthy people. This knowledge led me to write a book about health pharmacology,* in which alimentary pharmacosanation substances are examined along with actual medicines for healthy people. Bulk consumer food products, such as flour, vegetable oils, sugar and alcoholic drinks have an important place among the former. Particular attention should be paid to these products in that they have been selectively victimized by modern technology. With a persistence that could be better directed elsewhere, they are refined (once again to the advantage of the producers but to the detriment of man) by the removal not of harmful but of useful substances. This transformation results, for instance, in refined sugar or distilled alcohol revalling chemical reagents in purity. The only question is, why is it thought that man needs such purity?

The discovery of brown sugar's health-giving properties was not fortuitous. However, when my colleagues and I became conscious of the need for a pharmacology of health and began to formulate the issues, our investigations into brown sugar assumed even greater significance, and we ended up devoting a great deal of time and effort

---

* I.I. Brekhman: *Man and biologically active substances*, Nauka, Leningrad (1976) (R). I.I. Brekhman: *Man and biologically active substances. The effect of drugs, diet and pollution on health*, Pergamon Press (1980).

to them. Equally detailed studies will be made in turn of coarsely ground flour, unrefined vegetable oil and the complex of biologically active substances found in natural wines that protects man from the pernicious effects of pure alcohol. Let critics reproach us for engaging in a pharmacology of derivatives — or waste products! After all, Hans Selye gave us the splendid example of the 'pharmacology of filth' that lead to the discovery of the general adaptation syndrome.

I.I. Brekhman

Acknowledgements

We would like to express our gratitude to our coworkers in the Department of Physiology and Pharmacology of the Institute of Marine Biology, Far East Scientific Centre of the USSR Academy of Sciences; I.V. Dardymov, L.I. Dobryakova, M.A. Dyakova, L.N. Zharska, R.N. Lesnikova, S.Ye. Lee, N.Ya. Stasenko, E.I. Khasina and others for their great help in the research on the biological activity of brown sugar.

The study would have been less comprehensive but for the ready response to our call by scientists from other institutes. For their great contribution to our knowledge of brown sugar we thank Prof. K.A. Meshcherskaya and Dr. V.A. Shibanov (Vladivostok Medical Institute); Dr. S.B. Golikov (Far East Technical Institute of the Fishing Industry); Candidate of Biology P.S. Zorikov (Mountain-Taiga Station of the Far East Scientific Centre, USSR Academy of Sciences; Candidate of Chemistry A.A. Semenov (Irkutsk Institute of Organic Chemistry of the Siberian Section, USSR Academy of Sciences); Prof. S.I. Zolotukhin and scientific worker V.F. Kremnev (Medical Faculty, Patrice Lumumba University of Peoples' Friendship, Moscow); Prof. Ya.A. Fedorov, Candidate of Medicine G.V. Filin and scientific worker N.V. Kaliberdin (Odessa Medical Institute); and Candidate of Medicine A.L. Vovsi-Koshteyn (High-Altitude Medico-Biological Research Laboratory, Tadzhik SSR Academy of Sciences, Dushanbe). We were greatly helped by V.N. Teodorovich, chief of the Main Directorate of the Sugar Industry, RSFSR Ministry of the Sugar Industry.

We are extremely indebted to V.N. Zharsky, Director of the Maritime Sugar Combine, without whose active participation and support this work would not have been possible.

CHAPTER 1

Health

Health is Nature's great gift. Man has received from Nature a surprisingly perfect structure enclosed within the contours of his body. Even more surprising is the extent of man's powers of resistance to life's hardships — for instance, to cold and heat, wounds and poisons — and his ability to cope with fear and emotional shocks, hunger and disease. However, not all people have the same gift of health; many squander it profligately, with the result that it deteriorates as the years go by and illnesses occur. Nearly everyone unites two opposite poles in his make-up — health and illness. In practical terms very few people enjoy perfect health, the majority live in what has been called the third or intermediate state, between good and bad health. Moreover, the bodies of sick people also resist illness, the outcome depending on the extent of their reserves of health.

From earliest times man has had to counter disease, has had to strive to save himself from its ravages and recover his health. This was the origin first of the practice and then the science of medicine. Despite this, from its very beginnings and throughout the centuries medicine has reflected the duality of the health-illness concept. Every medical doctrine consists of two parts: the science of health and the science of illness (including its treatment). But the more medical science has discovered about illness and the more perfect its methods of treating disease have become, the more promising the way of achieving health by curing disease has seemed. Medicine has grown increasingly therapeutic, overspecialized and hospital-oriented,[1] ever more of a paradigm, whose adherents are convinced that in the final analysis therapeutic medicine will solve all the problems. However, this has not been the case. Despite the successes of medical science and the expenditure by Western nations of an ever greater proportion of their gross incomes on treating the sick, the incidence of illness and economic loss on medical grounds have remained high and, according to some indicators, are even rising.[2] A case in point is the USA, where a sharp increase in the proportion of the national income spent on

5

health care over the past 20 years has failed to produce a proportional fall in the death rate and an increase in the average life span.[3] Neither social nor medical measures, then, have had the anticipated effect of preserving the health of the general population. The reason for this is that medicine, although pursuing one aim, that of health, in effect resolves a completely different one, the treatment of disease. But the treatment of disease only sometimes produces health, and by controlling or removing disease one might say it does so by negative means. As J.S. Chapman writes: 'Medicine has indeed very little knowledge of or techniques for production of health as a positive activity . . . It is a curious phenomenon that while in human biology we have remained preoccupied with morbid processes, we have simultaneously produced animal husbandrymen and agronomists.[4] The same argument was put forward much earlier by the great medical theoretician I.V. Davydovsky: 'Isn't it time', he asked, 'to make the healthy individual the object of medical research and not the subject of attempts to find this or that illness in him?'.[5]

It is of the utmost importance that not one but two different goals are clearly realized: the first is health, the second is the treatment of illness. These targets are closely interlinked. But the strategy, tactics and 'technology' of successfully reaching both targets presupposes two different scientific solutions and two separate systems to be implemented in practice.

Health is one of the things we value most. As with any other material or spiritual value, personnel and matériel are required to attain ('generate') it. Take away any of the elements of this triad of relationships and the result you will get is nil. To begin with let us see how fully this triad has been realized in modern medicine. The goal is the treatment of illness; the facilities, or resources, are represented by the entire arsenal of medicine (the matériel); the personnel, or manpower, is the doctor who knows how to cure disease. The triad is complete, thereby satisfying logically medicine's stated objective. And millions of ill people are freed from their ailments. But is mankind the healthier for all this? Illnesses leave an aftermath, chronic diseases are reaching epidemic proportions. And what is the position with regard to the health of healthy people?

Let us examine the triad in which health forms the objective. The facilities are also well known: personal physical and mental hygiene; a daily routine (of work, rest and food); motor activity (physical exercise including sport); rational nutrition, including useful biologically active substances, medicinal among others. The personnel would be health specialists who in Chapman's opinion should not be trained at medical institutes but at establishments of a completely different type giving no place to pathology in the curriculum.[4] Health as an aim in its own right is not pursued by medicine (which is excessively preoccupied with another activity, namely treating the sick) or by any other specialized spheres. Of course health does depend to some extent on those who teach schoolchildren and students, on nutrition specialists, on those who provide specialized instruction in physical exercise and sport, and many others besides. But the relevance of what each specialist has to teach about health is secondary to his or her individual and specific aims. Such people are not united by the common purpose of creating health. Thus there are no health specialists, and what is more people are often not aware of the requirements that are involved (we shall examine this aspect in more detail shortly). To all intents and purposes, then, each of the three elements of the triad is missing. So is it any wonder that the health of mankind leaves much to be desired?

Viewed from a more general viewpoint, it is evident that there is no science that deals with man, modern man, in his entirety. Mankind has virtually surrendered himself to a medicine that examines him through the prism of pathology. A science of health should become an integral component of the science of man. We are not talking here about a medical science but an entirely new science, formed at the point where ecology, biology, medicine, nutrition, psychology, education and several other sciences converge. This science of health might be called 'valeology', from the Latin word 'valeo', meaning 'I am well', 'I am fit'. An altogether new kind of educational establishment, along with the requisite laboratories and scientific research institutes of valeology, would be needed to train specialists (scientists and practitioners). One can even foresee a time when many countries will have both a ministry of health and a ministry of medicine (the preservation of health through the treatment of illness).

It would be impossible even to list here the multitude of problems which valeology would be called on to solve. We will dwell on just two of them. The first, the pharmacology of health, has already been formulated to some extent. The second, the psychology of health, needs to be stated and defined as a matter of the utmost urgency.

In I.I. Brekhman's book *Man and biologically active substances. The effect of drugs, diet and pollution on health*,[6] it was proposed that pharmacology be divided into two parts — pharmacotherapy and pharmacosanation (the pharmacology of health). Pharmacosanation involves the science of the action of biologically active substances entering the body in the form of food or medicines that forestall illness, greatly increase resistance to various adverse factors, and restore to normal changes in body functions.

The first and principal medicine of pharmacosanation is rational nutrition (alimentary pharmacosanation), that is, a food intake in balance with regard to the main food substances (proteins, fats and carbohydrates), and containing vitamins, minerals and other biologically active substances which ensure an adequate range of 'structural' information (see Chapter 2). Together with the calorie content, the quantity of the structural information should be a second and essential integral criterion of food products and intake. Food as a biologically significant signal is always concomitant with a corresponding form of substance and energy. This dualism between information and energetics may be regarded in the light of the complimentarity principle formulated by Niels Bohr for particle-wave dualisms in physics.[7] And Bohr's words 'Contraria non contradictoria sed complementa sunt' ('opposites are not contradictory but complimentary') are equally applicable to food.

The second group of pharmacosanation substances consists of medicines that can be used by healthy individuals for specific purposes. These are primarily the adaptogens (ginseng, eleutherococcus and so forth),[8] which increase the body's overall nonspecific resistance, enabling it to respond more stably to stress.[9] To this category belong certain tranquillizers, for instance natural preparations from *Rauwolfia serpentina* Benth, and the horns of European reindeer *Saiga tatarica*,[10] which are capable of helping millions of people to cope with the pressures of modern living. Among the stimulants, caffeine-containing and similarly acting drinks, and certain synthetic substances (amphetamine, for example) may be assigned to pharmacosanation medicines, but the synthetic substances should only be prescribed in special circumstances. Vitamins are extremely important, not only in their specific roles but also as medicines for nonspecific prophylaxis,[11] i.e. as anti-atherosclerotic, hypotensive and anti-carious substances; as preparations that regulate sleep and appetite, thereby, helping, for instance, to break the habit of smoking or to deal with menopausal problems; and as medicaments that increase the span of active life. In addition there is the entire range of medicines taken by healthy individuals in order to avoid illness.

It should be emphasized that pharmacosanation's aims and medicines fully conform to scientific forecasts in the fields of biology and medicine in which the overwhelming majority of the tomorrow's medicines will be aimed not at the sick but at the healthy.[6]

Following the traditional belief that the road to health lies in treating disease, mankind has pinned its highest hopes on the natural sciences, and above all on molecular biology. Yet all the fruits of current and future research will only be beneficial provided our way of life and conduct (our 'health behaviour') are conducive and not destructive to health. What good are the very best medicines for curing illness, let alone prophylactic medicines for the healthy, if people neglect their regimen of work, rest and food, take little exercise, smoke and drink to excess? Does science develop, and industry produce medicines only to counteract the effects of man's laziness and his bad habits?

Of course it is a sad paradox that the vast majority of people know, know only too well, what is good and what is bad for their health. They know but do not follow sensible rules. It is indeed a riddle on a global scale that as far as their own health is concerned modern educated man behaves worse and less rationally than his ancestors. We have to face the fact that the problem of people's health, a peculiarly human conundrum, is very largely psychological in its origin. Hence the crying need to elucidate the problem of psychology of health as an essential first step in the development of a concept of heath instruction.

It is common knowledge that actual experience is the best guide and that people turn to the experience of their fathers and elders in order to shorten the path of learning, but because they pay little heed to their prophets, spontaneous prohibitions or taboos have come into being. With the emergence of religions many rules of hygiene were transformed into 'divine' laws, later consolidated in various sacred books, the Bible, the Koran and others, in the form of diverse religious precepts and proscriptions. Even when observance of these was not very strict they still served a purpose. Contravention of a precept was a 'sin', with both the clergy and the community at large holding the whip hand over 'sin'. In this indirect rather than direct way, through the interpretation of transgression, a person's health was taken out of his hands and fell under the control of public opinion. Prohibitions may have lost some of their force in today's world but public opinion has not; on the contrary, the general level of education has risen and people have become more aware. For these reasons the main effort to impress a system of health instruction should be directed via the intellect. It was precisely this way of protecting people from stress that Selye chose in recommending 'altruistic egotism'.[9] But the road to hell is paved with good recommendations as well as with good intentions. What can be done to ensure that people follow this advice, so that knowledge is turned into action?

The Universal Declaration of Human Rights and other international and national documents set forth a person's rights to a certain standard of living and to medical services necessary for the maintenance of health and the well-being of himself and his family.[12] It would be very useful if similar documents were to define with equal clarity a person's obligations towards his own health and the health of those close to him. After all, health is national property as well as a private possession. However, unless people are made aware of their responsibilities in this matter and are actively involved we are unlikely to see an overall improvement in the health of Western nations.

Mind you, this is not to say that people do not understand the importance of health and do not know how to value it. But most people only set a real value on their health when it is seriously threatened or has deteriorated significantly. At that point, and only then, they become motivated to seek a cure for their illness and to re-cover their health. And is there evidence that healthy people are motivated to keep themselves in good health? The answer is, not much. Even those who have to pay vast sums to be treated for their illnesses (and what about that for an incentive to look after yourself!) are almost as little concerned about their health as those who receive free medical treatment. Just what motivates people to take care of their health is a very complex issue and needs to be investigated by scientists who are also qualified as psychologists.

We need, for instance, to find out why people are not naturally motivated to eat sensibly and take exercise, and why the motivation to consume alcohol or to smoke persists in spite of their harmful effects on the body. The probable reason is that good or bad effects are not felt immediately but only several years or even decades later. With regard to nutrition there is some feedback from research, but it takes a very long time for the results of research to percolate through society. The explanation is that the mechanisms of biochemical adaptation oppose clinical manifestations of nutritional imbalances (deficits or excesses of nutrients) and pronounced disturbances or disease arise only after the adaptation reserves have become depleted.[13] A similar phenomenon is observed with chronic consumption of alcohol and heavy smoking over a long period.

The situation would presumably be different if the effects of physical exercise, for instance, were immediate and tangible on the basis of both subjective criteria (which are not unimportant) and objective criteria. Of great interest in this context is the system of aerobics devised by the American doctor Kenneth H. Cooper incorporating a 12-minute test which provides an effective means of monitoring one's own performance.[14] Here is an example of the operation of positive feedback. A rapid negative feedback reaction during exposure to insidious influences of a harmful nature, such as alcohol and nicotine, would be an important factor in controlling desire. With this end in view one can easily foresee the routine addition of harmless

years the excessive intake of fats and other foods rich in cholesterol was regarded as the prime dietary cause of hyperlipidaemia and atherosclerosis among other risk factors. The majority of writers in the field now consider that the excessive consumption of carbohydrates, particularly refined sugar, is the leading dietary factor.[40] Yudkin's studies showed that the average daily sugar intake of patients with coronary and peripheral vascular disease is higher (113 g and 128 g, respectively) than that of the healthy subjects in the control group (58 g).[26] Yudkin's book and Robinson's article[41] list several other illnesses linked with the over-consumption of white sugar and other refined carbohydrates. Among these are gastrointestinal disorders including chronic constipation, leading to varicose veins, dyspepsia, stomach and duodenal ulcers, diseases of the liver and bile duct, and even cancer of the colon. Caries occupies a prominent place in the pathology detailed. But perhaps the most universal consequence of eating too much sugar and other refined carbohydrates is a lowering of the general level of health, a fall-off in the body's reserves, and a weakening of the ability to adapt physiologically. One thing is certain, white sugar is unhealthy sugar.

CHAPTER 4

Attempts to Solve the Sugar Problem

The preceding chapter was given the same title as Yudkin's book *Pure, white and deadly*. But the book is subtitled *The problem of sugar*, and certainly the author of this serious, interesting and indispensable work has highlighted the problem as no-one else has done, stressing its great biological, medical and social importance. Indeed, (apart from pure alcohol) is there any other mass-consumed foodstuff that is so harmful to man? Yet Yudkin's book gives no suggestions as to how we might deal with the problem of sugar. Listed below are some well known sugar substitutes and certain additives. But these have not resolved the problem. We have had centuries of experience with white sugar, and its use is now so commonplace that it is extremely difficult to take any steps against it.

There would appear to be a very simple and, in many respects, economically advantageous solution to the problem — get people to halve their white sugar intake. But it is equally apparent that this would be far from easy. Force of habit is extremely powerful and it is all too difficult to overcome the inertia of current industrial techniques for the production of confectionery, soft drinks and a host of other sugar-containing products.

The chief reason, of course, is human nature. Seen from a purely everyday human aspect sugar is much more than mere sweetness: it is ideal, calorie-filled, satisfying sweetness; it is tasty, satiety. Cakes, chocolate, ice-cream, various drinks and many other products and dishes would be quite unacceptable without sugar. Tea alone is drunk without sugar in some countries.

Some people started eating less sugar when accounts of its harmfulness first appeared. But these people were in a clear minority. Evidently the self-imposed reduction of daily amounts of refined sugar is as unattainable to some people as containing alcohol is to others. In the previous chapter we described the principle involved in the mechanism leading to the development of a craving for alcohol or sugar. The Japanese proverb about their wine *sake* could be rephrased to run:

28

'first man eats sugar, next sugar eats sugar, and then sugar eats man'. There is undoubtedly an underlying genetic factor involved in conditioning the craving people develop for sugar, and it deserves serious scientific study.

From the following figures it will be seen that sucrose (white sugar) is not the sweetest of the sugars:—

Comparative sweetness of different sugars[42]

Sugar	Comparative sweetness, %
Fructose	173
Invert sugar (mixture of glucose and fructose)	130
Sucrose	100
Glucose	74
Maltose	32
Galactose	32
Lactose	16

For many reasons, however, it is sucrose that has received preferential and widest utilization. The sweetest sugar is fructose, which is very widespread in nature. But what has probably happened is that the selection of cultivated sucrose plants has proved considerably more successful. It is not known how fructose would behave in the industrial sugar production process. Invert sugar is obtained during the industrial production of sucrose (white sugar). It is an unstable product and does not always conform to the same standards. As can be seen in the above table glucose and other sugars follow sucrose in the sweetness league.

For many centuries our forebearers satisfied their desire for sweetness with fruits, berries, melons, water-melons and other products of nature in a fresh, dried and sun-cured form. There was diversity in the range of sweet mixtures and foods in which, it goes without saying, sugar was not present because it did not exist or was scarce and expensive. Throughout the ages man's requirements have been met by his old friend honey. He has also helped himself to the sap of birches, maples and various other trees.

However, with the development of the mass production of sweets, confectionery, soft drinks, wines and other items, man's old standbys proved technologically uneconomic and so could not be widely utilized. Nonetheless when white sugar's negative qualities came to light interest was rekindled and several countries produced sweets and other foods containing, for instance, the natural juices of certain plants. Research has shown that birch sap, raspberries, strawberries and many other berries and fruits are full of the natural sugar xylitol, the taste of which is indistinguishable from sucrose. In one research project one half of a large group of subjects ate xylitol for two years and the other half ordinary sugar. It was found that the incidence of dental caries was nine times lower with xylitol than with sucrose. But xylitol is ten times more expensive than ordinary sugar, there are not the same abundant sources of the raw material as there are for cane and beet sugar, so it is scarcely feasible that this sugar will make much headway.

More promising, perhaps, is hesperidin, which American and Japanese researchers have extracted from the skins of mandarin oranges and grapefruit. By means of chemical reactions and bacterial ferments this bitter product is converted into a purified sweet substance, which when combined with a small amount of fructose yields a powder that readily dissolves in water and is suited in principle for use by the confectionery industry. Hesperidin's main asset is that it is 100 times sweeter than sugar and does not exceed it in calorie content. Consequently it introduces 100 times fewer empty calories into the body.

Something must be said about the hexahydric alcohol sorbitol, isomeric with mannitol (manna sugar), which is found in many fruits and berries. It is half as sweet as sucrose, well tolerated and in daily doses of 25−30 g does not increase blood sugar. It is used to make dietetic products for diabetics.

In enumerating natural sweeteners one should not omit to mention the roots of the liquorice plant (*Glycyrrhiza*), known to people for more than 5,000 years. The leaves of the Paraguayan shrub *Stevia rebaudiana* have long been used in South America as a tea sweetener and in the canning industry. Stevioside, a triterpene glycoside which is 300 times sweeter than sucrose, has been extracted from the leaves of this shrub but is not a permitted food additive. More recently it was established that the protein monellin, extracted from the berries of *Dioscoreophyllum cuminsii* [the serendipity plant − translator], is 2,000 times sweeter than sucrose. A similar protein, theumatin, has been isolated from the fruit of the West African plant *Thaumatococcus deniellii*, and it is 4,000 times sweeter than sucrose. The berries of the African plant *Synsepalum dulcificum* owe their sweetness to the presence of the glycoprotein miraculin. It is clear from the article by K.J. Parker[43] (that provided this information) and from other sources that the fruits and various parts of plants have been widely used by the local populations; however, the super-sweet substances isolated from them have not been deployed on a wide basis.

The story of synthetic sugar substitutes starts of course with saccharine. This substance was synthesized in 1879. Saccharine is 300 times sweeter than sugar but at the same time is bitter and leaves an unpleasant after-taste. Some 60 years later cyclamate was synthesized; it is only 30 times sweeter than sugar and its after-taste is less disagreeable.[44] Saccharine and cyclamate are used in the manufacture of food-stuffs. They give the body no calories but are not without significance (particularly in their decomposition products). At the end of the day they have not been used on a wide scale and have long been banned in many countries.

Yudkin is perfectly correct in surmising the possibility that saccharine and cyclamate (the same also applies to other sugar sub-stitutes) would reveal more of their negative aspects, and with greater definition, if taken in 'enormously unrealistic amounts' for as long as sugar.[26] In noting the negative characteristics of these sugar sub-stitutes, Yudkin calls attention to the main fact, which is that they are synthetic substances. This is virtually the same as the judgment passed by Commoner's third law of ecology,[45] which proclaims that the introduction of artificial substances into the body not occurring in nature is likely to be harmful. His warning, delivered against syn-thetic medicines, should be even more strictly heeded when foodstuffs and additives are involved.

White sugar is obtained from the sap of the sugar beet and the sugar cane which contains a great variety of diversified substances. These are almost all lost during the process of extracting white sugar from them. Most attention has been paid to the almost total loss of trace elements, particularly chromium, a deficiency of which upsets carbo-hydrate and lipid metabolism. The book *Minerals: Kill or cure*[46] cites calculations made by Schroeder to the effect that there are 1.59 micrograms of chromium in raw sugar, 1.19 in brown sugar, and 0 in white sugar. The same book gives figures showing that when chromium is added to food it improves the indicators for testing glucose tolerance in 40% of elderly people with moderate disturb-ance and in 50% of adults with incipient diabetes. Research findings indicate that the daily addition of chromium could show that the role of chromium is associated with a dietary factor which influences the body's tolerance to glucose and is a low-molecular, soluble and thermostable compound of chromium. This organic chromium compound is more readily assimilated by the body than inorganic chromium compounds and it has an insulin-stimulating effect.[17]

Chromium deficiency, particularly in refined sugar, is regarded as one of the most important causes of atherosclerosis. It has been noticed that the tissues of people dying of atherosclerotic complications contain significantly less chromium and manganese than the norm.[47] There is ample statistical data proving that a deficiency in these trace elements determines a greater prevalence of atherosclerosis.[48] In this connection attempts have been made to enrich sugar with one or more trace elements. Reports have also been made of the fortification of sugar with iron compounds combined with ascorbic acid.[49]

These and many other endeavours to enrich sugar with trace elements have not been widely publicized, presumably on account of the inefficacy of trace element additives. However, chromium and all the other trace elements in sugar-bearing plants are far from being the only substances in which white sugar is deficient. They and macronutrients have been taken up because it is comparatively easy to identify them in products and in animal tissues. Natural organic compounds are many times more complicated to study, although it would seem that they are precisely the ones present in an enormous range in the molasses which, as is well known, make one of the best feeds for agricultural livestock.

Not one of the measures described above has been introduced on a mass scale, nor has it solved the sugar problem, which continues to worry not only scientists, doctors and sugar consumers but also sometimes even sugar manufacturers. Yudkin tells how one sugar industrialist, convinced of refined sugar's harmfulness, proposed that a search should be made to find an antidote which would be added to sugar.[26]

A natural antidote of this kind should have several properties. The complex of biologically active substances needed for it should come from a plant product, be available in large quantities, and be administered with a sugar mixture possessing good taste qualities. Such a sugar additive must be completely harmless and able to counteract the negative characteristics of white sugar. We have been using additives of this kind extracted from the roots of eleutherococcus (*Eleutherococcus senticosus* Maxim.) and from the berries of schizandra (*Schizandra chinensis* [Turcs.] Baill.). Eleutherococcus, which has now become widely known and used on every continent, deserves special attention. In their mode of action medicines from the root of this plant have an invigorating, adaptogenic, antistress, antiatherosclerotic, antidiabetic (etc.) effect, diametrically opposed to sugar's negative one.[8] At our suggestion eleutherococcus and schizandra sugar has been made since 1976 in the Soviet union.[50] However, during the past six years these two sugar additives have only been manufactured in small amounts, and we do not yet have figures for the extent to which the substances extracted from eleutherococcus root and the juice of schizandra berries reduce sugar's harmful effect. What we do know is that when eleutherococcus sugar is taken for a long time it lowers the overall incidence of disease, including susceptibility to influenza. On the other hand, eleutherococcus extract also has this effect when taken on its own, without sugar. Nevertheless the idea of a natural antidote is an important approach as a feasible way of resolving the problem of white sugar. The possibilities for research in this field are vast. There are huge numbers of plants on the face of the earth, many of them well studied, which are utilized in food and for therapeutic purposes. Nor is it hard to come by plants so constituted as to substantially mitigate the harm caused by white sugar. But why adopt such a complicated procedure? Why refine sugar from the natural complex of biologically active substances in sugar beet or sugar cane, and add to sugar yet another complex which moreover must first be created? Would it not be simpler to add extracts of these sugar-bearing plants to sugar itself? But what is the point of adding them when you already have the mixture — in under-refined brown sugar? In the beginning there was nothing else, and it was only comparatively recently that the manufacturing process of white sugar was mastered. Yet it has not ousted brown sugar completely — even now many countries eat only brown sugar. But what do we know about it?

CHAPTER 5

What We Know About Brown Sugar

When we began our study of brown sugar we found that there was practically no information available about its biological action. The position has not altered even now. What little we have learnt has been gathered in this chapter.

It should be said at the outset that modern man is painfully ignorant both about white sugar and about its varieties. Some people think that the only sugar that exists is easily soluble and that it is a modern invention for modern man who is always in a hurry and never has time for anything. Most people have never seen a sugar loaf (sugar moulded into a conical shape and weighing 3 kg), and many people have forgotten the taste of chipped sugar held in the mouth while drinking unsweetened tea, and always taken in smaller amounts than when stirred in the cup. In some parts of Asia powdered sugar refineries make sugar in large granulated cubes.

White sugar is indeed a product of modern technology. It is a surprising instance of how a foodstuff with the purity of a chemical reagent comes to be manufactured in tens of millions of tons. In the pre-technological era, only 100 or less years ago, the bulk of manufactured sugar was unrefined. In modern technological terms, it was either raw sugar or varying degrees of under-refined, so-called brown sugar. This is also the situation today in many developing countries in Asia and Africa, where the overwhelming majority of people eat brown sugar. The industrialized nations of Europe and the Americas have white as well as brown sugar. It is sold in shops and served at table in cafes and restaurants. Brown sugar is generally believed to be tastier and to cause a better aroma in coffee than white sugar. It is an essential component of many cocktails. From his conversations with many individuals in several countries one of the authors concluded that most people cannot distinguish between white and brown sugar except by their colour and taste. Many of them think that as taste is the priority one can dismiss the 'little harm' done by the impurities of brown sugar.

In countries where white and brown sugar are both used, brown sugar is clearly at a disadvantage in the scant attention it receives from its producers. White sugar is always standardized, permeated with identical crystals or confined within the strictly geometrical planes of moulded lumps. Brown sugar comes in a great variety of colour, ranging from dark brown (in raw sugar) to yellowish. Raw sugar consists of crystals that vary enormously in size and the pieces are usually irregular in shape. Brown sugar is the Cinderalla of the sugar industry. It is called by even worse names — 'bastr' (from the word bastard, or illegitimate) — and is regarded as a low-quality sugar.

But this attitude to the dark aspects of sugar is not held everywhere. India, for instance, as it has done for many centuries, manufactures 'gur' or 'jaggery' (raw sugar), a substance made from the juice of either the sugar cane or of certain kinds of palms. Ranging in colour from dark brown to cream gur is also widely used today for making sweets, puddings, cakes and some drinks. Indians greatly value gur's taste and useful qualities, consume it both as a food and as a medicine.[30]

The industrialized nations of Europe and America have a very strange attitude towards brown sugar. They produce and sell it, they eat it with their meals, and at the same time they are uncomplimentary about it. Yudkin has headed one chapter of his book 'Brown is beautiful', but he has far more bad than good to say of brown sugar.[26] A person will be much healthier, Yudkin writes, if he uses only brown sugar and never eats any food containing refined sugar. Elsewhere the only good he sees in brown sugar is that since one cannot eat the same amounts of brown as white sugar its harmful effects will not be so great: Raw sugar, in his view, is a dirty material, and eating it does not supply a person with all the vitamins and minerals his body needs. Yudkin believes that brown sugar is as bad as white because it contains 90–95% sucrose; therefore it cannot be argued that refined sugar is 'unnatural' and raw sugar 'natural'. To say this, he writes, is about as sensible as saying that I am dressed if I am wearing all my clothes including my tie, but I am undressed if I take it off; a man without a tie cannot be considered undressed, but a tie is a very important item of dress and a person is not properly dressed without it.

As far as sugar is concerned, without the substances accompanying raw or brown sugar it is indeed nothing but 'undressed' sucrose. Just as 'undressed' is pure alcohol and the so-called chief active principle of a medicinal plant which has been extracted in a pure form. Together with virtually unclothed white flour they constitute man's most mortal enemies. And it is not by chance that some writers stress there is nothing 'pure' in nature. It is a fact that Nature greatly complicates everything she makes.

The time has now come to describe what brown sugar is, whether it is clean or dirty, and what this dirt consists of.

There are many plants in nature that contain large amounts of sugar, but only two of them, sugar beet and sugar cane, have proved their full economic worth in providing many tens of millions of tons of sugar to satisfy the requirements of the world's population. Sugar beet is cultivated in temperate zones, sugar cane is grown in southern latitudes.

Sugar, with a large number of impurities, is obtained when the raw material is crushed and sprinkled with water. After being boiled down and purified as well as crystallized to some extent, pulp sugar [bagasse] is produced. Dark yellow or brown in colour it contains about 1% water, is bitter to the taste and generally speaking is not used for food purposes. The raw sugar then goes to a sugar refinery, where it is melted, undergoes further purification and crystallization, and ends up in the complex production line as approximately 85% white sugar (product 1) and 15% of as yet unrefined products 2 and 3, which are recycled to be turned into white sugar. It is these bi- and tri-products which are usually called brown sugar. They, like raw sugar, consist of white sugar crystals coated with a thin layer of molasses. Thus it is not so much a tie, as a dressing-gown enveloping the entire body.

Yudkin[26] gives the following figures for the sucrose content of various industrial sugar products: raw sugar — 96%; tri-product — 86.3%; bi-product — 89.1%; and the main product (white sugar) — 99.1% (in white sugar the quantity of sucrose can reach as high as 99.75%, which means the virtual approximation of a foodstuff to a chemical reagent). The rest is comprised of the complex of natural biologically active substances present in the original raw material of sugar production. Obviously the percentage content of these substances is even greater in the molasses. Depending on their amounts, their 'dirt', one can differentiate between white (29% non-saccharides), green (33%), brown (47%) and feed (55% molasses). These figures were obtained during an investigation of the different kinds of molasses formed during the processing of raw cane sugar at the Ussurysk Maritime Sugar Combine (Maritime Province, USSR). The non-saccharide content may vary somewhat.

As Yudkin writes, brown sugar can be produced by cutting short the refining process or by adding molasses to white sugar. Brown sugar (a bi-product), which we have obtained from the Maritime Sugar Combine, has been the object of all our research.

In its external aspect brown sugar is a uniform crystalline sugar, yellow-brown in colour and sweet to the taste. It has a pleasant, specific after-taste and a slight, agreeable aroma. It dissolves fully in water giving a transparent tawny solution. The brown sugar we examined possessed the following variables:

Sucrose (minimum)	96.0%
Reductase (minimum)	0.13%
Water (minimum)	0.2%
Chromaticity, in Stammer units (minimum)	12

Before passing on to the chemical composition of brown sugar, or rather those substances which accompany the sucrose in it, let us examine data about the chemical composition of the chief sugar-producing plants — sugar beet (*Beta vulgaris*) and sugar cane (*Saccharum officinarum*). Without exception, studies of the chemical composition of these plants, grown in millions of tons, have been inadequate. More often than not food and medicinal plants have been approached from the viewpoint either of the so-called leading food substance or from the angle of the 'chief active principle'. Sugar beet and sugar cane are mostly valued for their sucrose. Much less attention has been paid to all the other substances they contain. However, the evidence in several reports[51] indicates that more than 50 biologically active substances have been discovered in sugar beet (somewhat fewer in sugar cane). But even these data are far from complete.

These plants, in which the sucrose content reaches 18—25% and over, incorporate smaller quantities of arabinose, sedoheptose, maltose, raffinose and other sugars. Organic acids play a large part in the non-sugar composition: adipic, hydrocaffeinic, glycolic, glutaric, glutaminic, citric, oxycaprilic, oxalic, malic, succinic and a number of others. Of particular interest is phytic acid (inositol hexaphosphoric acid), whose calcium-magnesium salt forms phytic — a plant medicine having a wide spectrum of prophylactic and therapeutic action.

Sugar beet contains oleanolic acid in the form of a glucoside known as 'Zuckerübensaponin', incorporating a glucuronic acid group as the sugar variety.

Sugar cane contains brassicasterol and sitosterol. Sitosterol is one of the best known anti-atherosclerotic medicines, while sugar beet contains spinasterol. Both plants incorporate a large variety of amino acids; leucine, isoleucine, tyrosine, glutamic acid, histidine, etc. Sugar cane has a 5—10% betaine content.

Certain purines (hypoxanthine, adenine, guanine, for example) also deserve attention. Various vitamins, especially the vitamin C and B groups, are represented as well. Examination of the sugar-producing plants' chemical composition shows that they contain no poisonous or powerfully acting substances which could pose a threat to man.

As was said above, sugar is made brown by a thin film of molasses which covers each sucrose crystal, P.E. Norris's book provides general information about the chemical composition of molasses.[30] Feed molasses, as supplied for animals, contains sucrose 30.08%), laevulose (8.76%), dextrose (13.06%), other carbohydrates and organic matter (13.20%), minerals (8.32%) and moisture (24.58%). The minerals comprise of a very large number of macronutrients and trace elements. According to Norris 13.2% of the organic matter is distributed as follows:

Gummy matter	2.70
Nitrogenous matter	1.06
Organic acids	3.20
Caramel and other products of decomposition formed the production of sugar	6.24
	13.20%

The relatively large amounts of organic acids and byproducts stand out.

There is very little published data on brown sugar's chemical composition. It has not been studied systematically. To some extent brown sugar may be regarded as sucrose contaminated by molasses, but there is no certainty that the thin coating on the sucrose crystals in brown sugar is identical with molasses as such. Nevertheless, all that is known about the chemical composition of molasses brings us closer to a knowledge of the chemical composition of brown sugar's non-sugar constituents. Although research into the chemistry of molasses has already been going on for many years the results have been fragmentary. Each group of chemists has only looked for what it has wanted to find in molasses. Not one systematic and comprehensive research project has been carried out into the chemical composition of molasses. Many works do not even make clear what kind of molasses has been studied and whether it has been obtained from sugar-beet or sugar-cane. Because of these circumstances we shall only summarize findings without giving references.*

---

* The authors have been greatly helped in compiling this information by Dr. A.A. Semenov of the Irkutsk Institute of Organic Chemistry, Siberian Branch of the USSR Academy of Sciences, to whom they express their gratitude.

The chemical composition of molasses, like that of any other product of plant origin, is extremely complex. The qualitative composition depends on the producer plant. It is probable that 'beet' and 'cane' molasses differ in their chemical constitution. The quantitative composition of molasses' components may be dependent on the place of origin, weather conditions, the genetic properties of the producer plant, fertilizers, and many other factors.

Apart from sucrose, molasses contains other monosaccharides, disaccharides and oligosaccharides of a heterocyclic nature, amino and carboxylic acids, complex organic pigments, and other chemical compounds. The majority of the compounds determined in molasses are of natural origin, that is they have been preserved in the molasses in the sugar cane. Other substances have been formed as a result of chemical changes occurring with natural compounds during the technological process. In addition molasses may have various impurities introduced during the different stages of processing the raw material.

Whatever its origin molasses contains large amounts of potassium and calcium salts. Sugar-beet molasses contains on average 100 mg/kg iron, 34 mg/kg zinc, and 18 mg/kg manganese. Lesser amounts of cobalt (0.59 mg/kg), boron, copper and molybdenum are present. Sugar-cane molasses is seen to contain chromium, lead, nickel, barium, molybdenum, silver, zinc, titanium and cobalt — all in quantities of less than 1 mg/kg. It contains large amounts of calcium, magnesium, silicon, iron and manganese. Also to be found in molasses of certain origins are cations of lead, cadmium, mercury and arsenic; moreover it has been noted that these elements accumulate during industrial processing. Examples of this are arsenic contents of 0.04 mg/kg, 0.27 mg/kg, and 0.04 mg/kg for sugar beet, molasses and white sugar respectively.

The principal inorganic anions are represented by chloride and sulphate. Phosphate, nitrate and nitrite are present only in negligible quantities.

Carbohydrates and substances containing carbohydrates feature largely. Different kinds of molasses have approximately the same amounts in them of glucose and fructose and varying amounts of other monosaccharides: glyceraldehyde, rhamnose, ribose, fucose, xylose, arabinose and galactose. Alpha-D-glucosaccharinic acid, 0.13% of which is found in sugar-beet molasses, is probably formed from glucose when the sugar-beet juice is converted into calcium hydroxide. All molasses have the disaccharide raffinose and the trisaccharide ketose in their composition. Oligosaccharides of the dextrin type and pectic substances have also been detected. The saponins make up 0.014% of the molasses. They are in smaller amounts in raw sugar and brown sugar. Phenol glycosides typifying ligno-carbohydrate complexes feature as well. The carbohydrate part of them is hemicellulose in character and incorporates aldobiuronic acids.

Molasses is rich in carbonium acids. Some of the acids identified in it are of bacterial origin and are accumulated during storage. The following classes of acids have been detected: fatty, monobasic, dibasic, unsaturated and hydroxy acids. Their total content is 5%. It is the fatty acids that are mainly responsible for the unpleasant aftertaste and smell of molasses. Acetic acid predominates in this class of acids, but all the other homologuous fatty acids are represented in smaller quantities, with straight and branched chains, ranging from formic to hexanoic. Oxalic and succinic acids are also present in small amounts. Lactic and the main acid in sugar-beet molasses, is related to the class of hydroxy acids. Its average content is 1.9%, while that of the other hydroxy acids, glycolic, malic and citric, is 0.3, 0.4 and 0.3, respectively. Among the organic acids in sugar-cane molasses unsaturated tribasic aconitic acid preponderates. It represents up to 40% of the total acids. Its calcium-magnesium salt imparts extra viscosity to the molasses.

Molasses incorporates up to 15% of nitrogenous matter, mainly amino acids. Of these, trimethylaminoacetic acid — betaine — is the principal non-sugar component of molasses. In content it is slightly in excess of 5%, though it can be considerably more. Molasses is also rich in glutamic acid (0.5%) and in pyrrolidine carboxylic acid (2.8%), a product of its cyclization. Other dominating free amino acids are: aspartic acid, leucine, isoleucine, valine, alanine and glycine. Sugar-beet molasses contains quite large quantities of γ-aminobutyric acid (0.3% maximum). Small amounts of polyethylene polyamines have been found. Heterocyclic compounds are also among the nitrogenous substances found in molasses. Some of them relate to melanoidins — coloured polymer components. Purines and pyrimidines have been detected among monomer heterocycles. Adenosine is their chief component and the adenosine content in dried molasses is 0.2–3%; it is comparatively easy to separate in its pure form. One of the substances giving molasses its smell is acetopyrrole.

Three groups of substances confer on molasses and brown sugar their tawny colour: the caramels, the melanoidins and the complexes of phenol and iron compounds. The chemical determination of all three has been poor on account of the complexity and variability of their composition. By caramels is meant the complex mixture of high-molecular compounds that are the products of the thermal conversion of sucrose. The melanoidins are nitrogenous compounds, products of carbohydrate reaction with amino acids and peptides. This chemical process, the Maillard reaction, leads to the formation of nitrogenous and oxygenous heterocycles, chief of which are several pyrroles and furans. Several methods have been proposed for dividing molasses' coloured compounds into fractions, and this has led to a general concept of the chemical nature of the melanoidins. They are a highly intricate conglomerate of substances whose molecular weight ranges from 700 to 50,000 and more. The polymer melanoidins have a long structure of molecules and are amorphous. The nitrogen and furan heterocyclic nuclei which form part of their constitution have side chains of residuary carbohydrates and amino acids.

The coloured substances of molasses have a technological origin; in other words they are absent in the initial plant material and are formed during processing. Consequently their composition depends not only on the quality and origin of the raw material but also on the characteristics of the technological regime.

The study of molasses' chemical composition is far from complete. To all intents and purposes the chemical structure of the melanoidins and the caramels is unknown, and likewise little is known about the composition of the phenols, whose iron-containing complexes are partially responsible for the dark colour of molasses. Some of them, such as bioxybenzaldehyde, vanillin and syringaldehyde are presumed to form when lignin is decomposed under the influence of $Ca(OH)_2$ and atmospheric oxygen during the refining of sugar. Numerous investigations reveal that molasses has no vitamin content. The list of chemical compounds discovered in molasses and other products of sugar refining grows longer all the time. For instance, in molasses and brown sugar from sugar cane considerable quantities have been found of ethyl phthalic acid ether and 2R-2-ethylhexanol, and also a mixture of lactones in which the lactone 2-methyl-D-ribonic acid predominates.

Dr. A.A. Semenov initiated systematic research into the chemical composition of brown sugar. According to his calculations, approximately 200 substances have been counted in brown sugar, detectable in amounts not less than several parts per thousand. He has developed an effective method of separating these fractions, discovering in the process two that had not been previously detected in either brown sugar or molasses.

The first of these substances (provisionally called 'matsiyef') was extracted from brown sugar's least polar fraction by means of column chromatography using silica gel, with subsequent high-vacuum distillation. This substance is a colourless, moderately viscous liquid with a boiling point of 155–160°C/0.05 mm and a refraction coefficient of n^2D-1,4850. Its molecular weight is 390 and the chemical composition is $C_{24}H_{38}O_4$. It was established that the substance was a natural complex of ethyl phthalic acid ether and 2R-2-ethylhexanol.

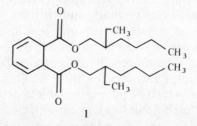

1

The content of this substance in brown sugar is variable, from trace amounts to total absence.

A.A. Semenov has separated a somewhat more polar group of substances which he has called a lactone fraction. This yielded a crystalline substance having the empirical formula $C_6H_{10}O_5$ which has been given the structure of a lactone of 2-methylribonic acid.

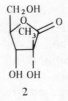

2

A description of the extraction of this substance from sugar-beet molasses has already been provided. It is formed as a result of the regrouping of glucose when acted upon by alkalis.

So far, as existing data makes clear, it has not been possible to find a substance or a group of substances representing brown sugar's 'chief active principle'. Maybe it will be found one day. If it is it will certainly consist of a fairly complex mixture of substances. One cannot exclude the possibility that the biological effects of brown sugar differ from those of white sugar by virtue of the entire complex of substances that accompany the sucrose. What is important in our view is the complexity of the diversified chemical composition which may be measured quantitatively by its structural information.

It is well known that molasses is an excellent feed for cattle — its many remarkable qualities are widely publicized by the suppliers of this produce. Emphasizing this point P.E. Norris, author of a book about molasses, asks: 'And if for animals, why not humans?'.[30] At the end of his book the writer gives a score or so of recipes of dishes and drinks made with molasses and recommends them as healthy food. However, he does not substantiate his claims scientifically. The fact is that data of this sort about the healthy properties of brown sugar and molasses is very hard to find. Literally the only findings are about its anticariogenic and antisclerotic action. They will be cited in the following chapters. Thus the conclusion to be drawn is that we know very little about brown sugar.

CHAPTER 6

The General Action of Brown Sugar in Animal Experiments Lasting up to 30 days

Brown sugar is not a medicament but a foodstuff. Millions of people eat brown sugar, and subjective reports of what they feel immediately after taking it or some time later are not likely to be very helpful. But this does not mean that there is no effect, only that the detailed experiments are necessary to demonstrate it. In this connection one cannot help recalling the history of ginseng (*Panax ginseng* C.A. Mey). There is of course good reason why this medicinal substance has been prized in the treasure-chest of oriental medicine for about 5,000 years. Had the favourable action claimed for ginseng not been genuine, it would have sunk into oblivion like so many other medicines have. Yet when scientists did get round to studying ginseng's effects, for a long time they obtained only negative results. It failed to act in experiments on healthy animals at rest or on their isolated organs. This gave rise to scientific myths about ginseng's ineffectiveness, which did not, however, succeed in toppling its legendary reputation.

Ginseng did at last reveal its secrets when one of the authors of the present book took a step off beaten track of pharmacological experiment. It was found that in animals compelled to carry out muscular work or subjected to various unpleasant stimuli ginseng raises the body's physical potential, increasing its overall nonspecific resistance. As a result 30 years have seen the accumulation of a great amount of experimental and clinical material on a group of medicines which have been called adaptogens. Recently we proposed a new term for these preparations, that of 'staminators', derived from the word 'stamina'.[52] Investigations of several other plants in the same Araliaceae family led to the discovery of eleutherococcus (*Eleutherococcus senticosus* — Maxim) which has surpassed legendary ginseng. It is against this background that studies have been made of the non-ossified horns ('panti') of the spotted deer (*Cervus nippon*), the European reindeer (*Rangifer tarandus*) and other kinds of deer.[53] At present we are investigating extracts with a similar action from a number of species of marine invertebrates.[54] Siberian researchers have recommended that extracts of the pink rodiola (*Rhodiola rosea* L.)[55] and certain other plants should also be classed as adaptogens. This group of medicaments, particularly eleutherococcus, play a leading part in the medicines of health pharmacology or pharmacosanation.[6]

Experiments to determine the effect of such substances on human or animal work capacity have been a touchstone and the first step along the lengthy path from ginseng to marine invertebrates. Our many years of research and the findings of many other scientists have convinced us that work capacity is an important integral indicator, an extremely sensitive one, of how the body feels, whether well or ill. The various aspects of physical and mental work capacity offer very promising prospects of research. But a prerequisite for screening and the preliminary testing of medicines or investigating the harmful effects of industrial poisons is a methodology based on the use of small laboratory animals. To this end we were one of the first to employ swimming by white mice,[56] but this was not wholly satisfactory and we were obliged to look for alternative test methods.

In 1963 we proposed a new method of registering dynamic work to the point of exhaustion using white mice. It involved the use of an original piece of equipment, which compelled the mice to run up a rope moving vertically downwards (an 'endless rope').[57] We found the method extremely reliable and sensitive, and it was used in our laboratory for about 20 years, as well as in many other laboratories. Its special merit was that it enabled us to determine the biological activity of the individual glycosides of ginseng, eleutherococcus and of substances isolated from a series of other plants. One great advantage of the method was that it only necessitated the use of milligrams of the test substances. It is of course due to this method's exceptional sensitivity that we discovered brown sugar's biological activity. It happened by accident and this is how.

In the course of a test on the sensitivity and reliability of the results obtained by this method, some granulated sugar that had been bought and ground into powder was included as a control standard in an investigated group of preparations of individual glycosides extracted from the root of a plant. Imagine our great surprise when this very ordinary foodstuff increased the work capacity of mice to a level comparable with summed extracts from several plants. Naturally we first thought that the production of energy by the carbohydrate was responsible for this enhancement, but glucose in much greater amounts did not have a similar effect. It was then that we suspected the admixture of incompletely refined sugar — since the granulated sugar we had used was not outstanding in its snow-whiteness.

We lived through a very difficult time. It seemed as if our method might be at fault, and this threatened all the data we had hitherto obtained, and most of what had been published as well. Then we tested several samples of chemically pure sucrose. In all cases the result was negative. Not only pure white but also 'dirty' glucose specimens, tawny and even dark brown in colour, proved to be inactive. It became clear that the source of the first sugar's biological activity lay in the impurities that remained as a result of incomplete purification during the refining process. We were pleased that not only had our method not misled us, but it had actually revealed the biological activity of the small traces of substances that accompany sucrose.

What more natural, then, than that we should visit a sugar refinery to obtain samples of brown sugar varying in degrees of refinement? An examination of brown sugar (products 2 and 3) showed that the higher the content of substances accompanying sucrose, the greater the brown sugar's activity: beet and cane brown sugar are roughly equal and only two to three times less active than ginseng and eleutherococcus root liquid extracts (Table 1).

Table 1. The effect of different kinds of sugar on the work continuity of mice
to complete exhaustion in stimulating units of action (SUA)

Plant	Foodstuff (preparation)	Content of substances accompanying sucrose, %	Number of SUA in 1 g	
			Product (preparation)	Substances accompanying sucrose or dry residue of preparation
Sugar beet	White sugar (product 1)	0.25	0	0
	Brown sugar (product 2)	10.9	25	230
	Brown sugar (product 3)	13.7	31	226
Sugar cane	Sucrose (pure for analysis)	0.1	0	0
	Brown sugar (product 2)	10.9	27	247
	Brown sugar (product 3)	13.7	28	204
Ginseng	Extract 1:1	—	67	670
Eleutherococcus	Extract 1:1	—	56	957

In the course of travels abroad one of the authors collected samples of brown sugar from a number of countries.[58] It was found that their biological activity varied in its stimulating action within narrow limits (Table 2). It transpired that the absence in some cases of a correlation between biological activity and the concentration of the substances accompanying sucrose depended on the varying extent to which brown sugar had been refined in the different countries.

Table 2. The biological activity of brown sugar samples from different countries in stimulating units of action (SUA)

Country	Content of substances accompanying sucrose, %	Number of SUA in 1 g	
		Brown sugar	Substances accompanying sucrose
USSR	10.9	27	247
USA	6.8	55	823
Great Britain (demerara sugar)	10.3	33	320
France	2.0	23	1150
Sweden	3.9	28	720
Denmark	3.5	31	890

As was pointed out in the previous chapter, brown sugar is a product consisting of white sugar crystals coated with a thin layer of molasses. In the process of producing and refining sugar four kinds of molasses (white, green, brown and feed) are obtained, varying in their sucrose content (Table 3). The less sucrose there is in molasses, the

Table 3. The biological activity of different kinds of molasses in stimulating units of action (SUA)

Molasses	Content, %		Number of SUA in 1 g	
	Sucrose	Substances accompanying sucrose	Molasses	Substances accompanying sucrose
White	71	29	50	172
Green	67	33	55	166
Brown	53	47	77	164
Feed	43	55	117	213

greater the amount of the substances accompanying sucrose. Research has shown that with an increase in the content of these substances there is a proportional increase in the SUA in 1 g of molasses. Data on the biological activity of 1 g of the substances accompanying sucrose is not so strictly dependent on their percentage content. It must be assumed that different kinds of molasses have substantial qualitative differences in their chemical composition, depending upon whether the content of the active and non-active substances is greater or lesser. A comparison between the activity of the substances accompanying sucrose in brown sugar (Table 1) and different kinds of molasses (Table 3) indicates that in general it is most likely to be a complex of substances closely allied in composition.

Attempts to equate brown sugar's activity with chromium and other trace elements contained in it have not proved successful to any extent. Information, which is far from complete, about brown sugar's chemical composition (see Chapter 5) is evidence of the presence in it of a large variety of potentially biologically active organic compounds. It also remains to be elucidated what contribution is made to the biological activity of molasses (and, correspondingly, of brown sugar) by the Maillard substances,[59] which form as a result of the condensation of carbonyl sugar groups with amino groups of amino acids in the process of converting and storing intermediate sugar products.

We examined the products of the division of molasses into two fractions: the Maillard substances and the complex of substances of natural origin.[59] We discovered that the activity of 1 g of the substances accompanying sucrose in molasses was 280 SUA, 1 g of the Maillard products was 58 SUA, and 1 g of the complex of substances of natural origin was 146 SUA. Thus although the Maillard substances contribute, the biological activity of molasses (and, correspondingly, of brown sugar) is determined to a large degree by the complex of substances of natural origin from sugar beet or sugar cane that have remained in these products.

Given that stress is inseparable from life itself, what, we wondered, would be the effects of comparable sugars on stress resistance in animal experiments?

A research project was carried out using 246 female white rats, weighing 140–170 g and divided into four equal groups. One group of rats was not subjected to stress (norm), while the other three groups were subjected to stress in accordance with the method proposed by our laboratory. The animals were hung for 18 hours by the fold of skin on the back of their necks. For one week prior to this isotonic saline (control), or 15 g/kg of a sucrose solution or a solution of the same amount of brown sugar was injected daily into the rats' stomachs.

The results showed that sucrose had very little effect on the amount of stress ('stress index' 9, compared with 7 in the control group (see ref. 60 — Table)). The substances concomitant with sucrose prevented a similar effect on the same amount of sucrose contained in the injected dose of brown sugar (the 'stress index' was 7, as in control). All the kinds of molasses examined had some anti-stress effect (see ref. 61 — Table).

Stress induces several marked biochemical changes. Changes in the sugar level, β-lipoproteins, deoxycorticosteroids in the blood and, especially, in liver glycogen were repeatedly used by us while studying the anti-stress action of eleutherococcus and the other adaptogens. From the findings of our colleagues I.V. Dardymov and E.I. Khasina, brown sugar is also seen to be an effective anti-stress agent in experiments of this kind, but it required the preliminary insertion by probe into the rats' stomachs of daily doses of 15 g/kg for a fortnight. Then the rats were suspended by the skin on the back of their necks for 24 hours.

This powerful stress effect produced in the control a definite increase in the discharge of deoxycorticosteroids into the blood, an increase in the blood content of sugar and β-lipoproteins, and also a reduction in the glycogen content of the liver. After white sugar had been administered for a fortnight the stress pattern was approximately the same. Brown sugar provoked less pronounced signs of stress (Figure 1) (see also ref. 62 — Table).

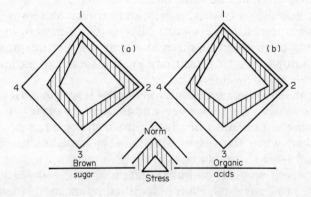

Figure 1. The influence of a preliminary fortnight's administration of brown sugar (15 g/kg) or a sum of organic acids (70 mg/kg) on specific signs of stress, expressed in indirect (1 — blood sugar, 2 — blood β-lipoproteins, 4 — blood deoxycorticosteroids) or direct percentages (3 — liver glycogen) (63 — Table).

When the above results were discussed it was suggested that organic acids, a major portion of which form the non-saccharide complex of the biologically active substances of brown sugar, were chiefly responsible for brown sugar's anti-stress and other effects. A factor that had to be taken into consideration was that organic acids have a central role in cell metabolism. They serve as an energy source — they are substances for the synthesis of carbohydrates, amino acids and lipids. They can participate in the formation of $NADH_2$ and $NADPH_2$, increase the content of the oxidized forms of co-ferments, and, in the final analysis, may change the direction of the metabolic flow in the cell and at the level of the whole body.

A mixture of oxalic, malic, succinic, glutamic, citric and glycolic acids was made from commercial samples using the amounts found in brown sugar. Experiments were carried out, similar to those described, in which daily doses of 70 mg/kg of this mixture of organic acids was fed into the rats' stomachs for a fortnight. The amount was exactly the same as in the 2.25 g of brown sugar which had been fed to rats weighing 150 g (15 g/kg). We hoped the mixture of organic acids would produce an effect but we did not expect that their anti-stress action would be the same as in the experiments with brown sugar (Figure 1) (see also ref. 63 — Table). The results provide food for speculation about the role of organic acids in brown sugar's prophylactic effects. However, data are needed on the other effects of white and brown sugar before a final assessment can be made.

R.L. Hays and his coworkers discovered that[64] rats fed exclusively on sucrose became pregnant at the same time as did the control rats (fed normal amount) but the number of implantation sites was reduced, as was the case with ovariectomized rats. Moreover, if the diet of sucrose was continued almost all the foetuses were lost but the mother rats themselves all survived — yet another demonstration of the well known greater sensitivity of the foetus to various adverse factors.

Professor A.P. Dyban and his co-authors[65] repeated Hays's experiments and established that when rats are kept on sugar and water, the subdivision and migration of the zygote in the oviducts occur normally. But then when the blastocysts failed to implant, all the embryos died on the 14th–15th day.

Our research was carried out on rats weighing 180–230 g. Female rats in the pro-oestral stage were identified by means of vaginal smears and placed on male rats at 1700 hours. In the morning vaginal smears were again taken and examined, this time for the presence of spermatozoa. The day on which spermatozoa were found in the smear was counted as the first day of pregnancy. Then the rats were divided into three groups and for the next 20 days of pregnancy 90% of the calorific value of the food they were given consisted of granular feed (control), white or brown sugar. The remaining 10% was supplied by a boiled hen's egg. On the 21st day of pregnancy all the rats were killed and on autopsy calculations were made of the number of brown bodies, implantation sites, dead foetuses and haemorrhaged foetuses. Pre-implantation and post-implantation loss was determined on a percentage basis.

As the results obtained show (Table 4), white sugar sharply increased the embryonic, post-implantation death rate, reduced the average number of live foetuses of each female rat and their median weight,

Table 4. The effect of white and brown sugar on the reproduction of female white rats.

Indicators	90%* feed pellets (control) + 10% boiled hen's egg	90% white sugar	90% brown sugar
Number of rats	29	30	27
Pre-implantation embryo loss, %	12.9 ± 2.9	13.4 ± 2.3	5.5 ± 2.4 p = 0.01
Post-implantation embryo loss, %	5.4 ± 1.7	18.3 ± 4.0	7.0 ± 1.7 p = 0.01
Total embryo loss, %	18.1 ± 3.5	31.7 ± 4.2	12.5 ± 2.2 p = 0.001
Total number of dead fetuses	–	20	–
Total number of live fetuses	8.6 ± 0.70	6.8 ± 0.73	8.0 ± 0.76
Average fetal weight, in g	3.8	2.4	2.8
Total number of haemorrhaged fetuses	7	53	17

* Percentages expressed by calorie content

and markedly increased the number of haemorrhaged foetuses. In this group alone it was found that there were 20 dead foetuses. Brown sugar more than halved the pre-implantation loss rate, even when compared with the control group, and in all other indicators yielded better results than white sugar.

Thus the experiments described in this chapter show that brown sugar and molasses increase the work continuity of white mice to complete exhaustion, even in a single dose, and that they heighten the body's resistance to stress; in addition, brown sugar reduces the toxic effect of sucrose. However, all the data were obtained from experiments in which rats received white or brown sugar for periods of not more than a month, which is only 1/25 of a average life of the rat. Sugar, on the other hand, is eaten by people throughout their lives. Therefore more prolonged experiments were carried out, as will be described in the following chapter.

CHAPTER 7

Brown Sugar's General Action in Prolonged Animal Experiments

Despite the details given in the last chapter concerning the positive influence of brown sugar on animals' work capacity, their resistance to stress and the absence of immediate toxicity, these findings do not resolve the main task of research on brown sugar, which in our view is to clarify the question as to whether brown sugar is harmless when taken over a long period — even throughout the animal's life.

However paradoxical it may seem at first sight, our data concerning the increased work capacity of animals given brown sugar turned out to be an additional argument in favour of the need for prolonged experiments. In fact, when a person consumes 100 g of brown sugar in 24 hours he obtains a quantity of biologically active substances having an activity of 2,500 SUA (corresponding to an activity of 1 g of 25 SUA). This total amount of activity corresponds to 37 g of ginseng root (Table 1), which is the amount known to have caused severe poisoning when taken after a single dose.[66] It is shown in practice that brown sugar may be eaten every day in these doses for many years without fear of poisoning. The reason lies in the different nature of the complex of active substances in ginseng and brown sugar. However, this is not a unique phenomenon: an increase in work capacity commensurate with the action of ginseng may be obtained from very small doses of amphetamine, although the latter is completely unsuited for repeated dosage, especially daily, but even weekly. By contrast, an extract from the roots of eleutherococcus, which is closely related in activity, is absolutely harmless. On a number of occasions people, who had been taking it daily for a decade or longer were tested with a single dose of 200 ml, equivalent to 11,200 SUA. Their response was entirely healthy, so stimulating units of action, which are important indicators of useful medicinal preparations and food products, cannot prognosticate toxicity and various other kinds of action.

As a matter of fact all the experiments conducted by us and by other researchers were designed to reveal the possible toxicity of brown sugar. We had not hoped to establish any actual positive effects when we speculated that brown sugar's innocuousness, combined with its good taste qualities might sufficiently justify its usage on a broad scale. Like Yudkin, we found it very hard to believe, that brown sugar was just as bad a food as white sugar.[26]

Since 1974 we and several other investigators have studied the possible toxicity or, more accurately, harmlessness of brown sugar compared with a chemically pure sucrose or white sugar. The sugars have been tested in doses ranging from 0.5 to 90.0 g/kg, and even when sugar has been substituted for an entire diet. The most frequent dosages used in the experiments were 2.0, 15.0, 30.0 and 50.0 g/kg, corresponding to 2, 15, 30 or 50% of the calorie value of an animal's daily food intake. Mainly rats, but also mice and rabbits, numbering over 3,500 animals, were used for the experiments, and they were given increased amounts of white or brown sugar for periods lasting from one week to two years and longer.

In one of our first experiments on 50 Wistar rats weighing 100—110 g, a comparison was made between the action of sucrose and brown sugar in a physiological dose of 2 g/kg and, in what seemed to us a decidedly large dose of 15 g/kg. The sugars were introduced into the stomachs of male rats by means of a probe every day for three months. The control rats were given an equal amount of an isotonic solution of sodium chloride. A blood sample was taken from the caudal vein before starting the experiment and again one month later. No differences were found between the rats in the three groups with respect to external appearance, behaviour and weight over the period of the experiment. Nor was any difference noted in the weight of the organs. Examination of both the red and white cell components of blood also failed to display any variations between the groups.

In another series of experiments, 2 g/kg of sucrose or brown sugar was administered to female rats for as long as six months. This had likewise no effect on the animals' condition and behaviour. Observations were made not only of the female rats but also of two successive litters (the females were sired by male rats fed their usual diet). As can be seen from Figure 2, brown and, to a lesser degree, white sugar reduced the interval of birth by 7—10 days. Moreover, rats in the first litter produced by females receiving white sugar weighed on average less than those in the two other groups. This difference was not seen at all in the second litter or had vanished within 30 days of birth. In the first and second litters both kinds of sugar increased the female rats' fertility by approximately equal amounts (20—24%). Subsequently, three female rats were taken from the first generation litter of each group, then, when each of them weighed 100 g, up to 2 g/kg of one or other sugar was administered every day for three months. These rats in their turn gave birth to a second ('sugar') generation of rats, in which the offspring produced by females given brown sugar were reliably shown to be heavier (Figure 2). There was no difference in fertility between rats on the sugar regimes and controls.

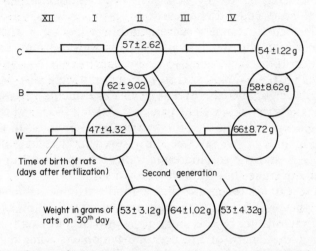

Figure 2. The influence of white (W) or brown (B) sugar on the birth periods of rats (black rectangles) and the average weight of the litter rats on the 30th day (encircled), compared with the control (C) in the first and second generations.

In the previous chapter we described our experiments showing that the substitution of white sugar for 90% of the calorie content of the diet fed to pregnant rats provoked a sharply expressed embryotoxic effect. The substances accompanying sucrose in brown sugar substantially weakened or completely removed the harmful effect of doses of pure sucrose. In view of this we thought it would be of very great interest to trace the trophic values of white and brown sugar under the stringent conditions attached to our research on the embryotoxic action.

For this purpose we employed Williams's method[67] of determining the trophic value of foods, in accordance with which male weaning rats were fed (*ad libitum*) a monodiet under conditions of what might be called alimentary stress. This American nutritionist considers that a food's fuel value can be judged on the basis of its ability to supply calories, and he provides a method for determining food's 'beyond-calorie' quality — its 'trophic' value. Male weanling rats were fed on a monodiet and observations were recorded of the number of the animals that perished during a 12-week period, the average life span of the survivors, and their median weight gain. An indication of the trophic value of a particular food (in all cases 10% of the fuel value of each monodiet was supplied by hen's eggs) was determined by a correlation between the average weight gain in the group of animals fed one of the monodiets and that of the rats in the control group fed a standard diet. According to the published findings, the trophic value of sucrose, glucose, and corn starch came to precisely zero. Nevertheless we still decided to compare sucrose and brown sugar in this exacting experiment with the standard diet used in our vivarium. Each group consisted of 14 rats averaging 45 g in weight. At the end of ten and-a-half weeks all the animals in the control group were alive and showed an average weight increase of 254 g. In experiments with sucrose 11 rats died, the survivors' weight gain was 9.0 ± 2.07 g, and the trophic value based on Williams's method indicated 3.5 units. In the brown sugar group only seven rats died, the survivors' weight gain came to 23.0 ± 3.7 g, and the trophic value indicator equalled 9 units. It is a very small difference but it favours brown sugar.

We were careful to ensure that a food's trophic value was calculated on the basis of only one indicator obtained in the experiment. The survival difference was not taken into account and in no way determined the length of life up to the moment when half the rats died (the 'half survival time'). This last indicator showed statistically significant differences in our two experimental groups (sucrose — 55.0 ± 2.4 days; brown sugar — 65.0 ± 3.3 days; $p = 0.034$).

We attempted to calculate the cumulative indicator of a food's trophic value on the basis of the above three characteristics. To do this we have represented the cumulative indicator of each food's trophic value as a vector, with its components constituting the parameter points of interest to us. In our case these are: survival, average half survival time (HST), and weight gain of the experimental animals

Q   — cumulative indicator of a food's trophic value,
x   — number of surviving rats,
x_1 — total number of rats in a group,
y   — average half survival time (HST) in days,
y_1 — total length of experiment in days,
z   — average weight gain of rats surviving in experimental group,
z_1 — average weight gain of control group.

To obtain dimensionless variables, we introduce the relationship of the corresponding parameters, in which case vector Q may be represented as three figures: $Q = (x/x_1 \quad y/y_1 \quad z/z_1)$ but the cumulative indicator of the trophic value may be given as the 'length' of this vector, calculated according to the formula:

$$Q = \sqrt{(x/x_1)^2 + (y/y_1)^2 + (z/z_1)^2}$$

Adapting this formula to our experiment, we obtain:

$$\text{sucrose } Q = \sqrt{(3/14)^2 + (55/74)^2 + (9/254)^2} = 0.77$$

$$\text{brown sugar } Q = \sqrt{(7/14)^2 + (55/74)^2 + (23/254)^2} = 1.01$$

In this way an answer is provided in relative units, taking into account the three research parameters. And in the same way it is possible to devise a formula based on a larger number of parameters that may be used to describe the trophic value of a foodstuff or a food diet. A defect of a cumulative indicator of a trophic value is that it cannot be calculated for the control group as it is impossible to determine the significance of 'y' for it — clearly, if the animals do not die it is not possible to calculate a HST. For this reason comparison with the control is impossible. But at the same time the method proposed by us of determining the cumulative indicator of a trophic value has the advantage that it permits comparison between different products or samples of one the same product closely related in trophic value (sugar, vegetable oil, flour, etc.); between those products differing in origin (brown beet and cane sugar; oil from the seeds of various plants); between the technology involved in extracting and the degree of refining; between the levels of preservation in storage; between culinary processing methods; and so forth. Williams and his co-workers, discounting small numerical values, confer the same zero rating on sucrose, glucose and starch, although, in their opinion, these products differ in all three of the research parameters. Had these researchers examined sugar they would also have obtained a zero rating for it. In the cumulative indicator of trophic value put forward by us, which takes a large amount of information into consideration, both types of sugar differ from each other. In the given instances one can hardly discount Q, equal to 0.77 for sucrose, because the value of the cumulative coefficient may be equated with an amplitude approaching the Figure 3. Consequently the comparatively small amount of substances accompanying sucrose in brown sugar has a trophic value. And if the sucrose only determines the calorie value, then the accompanying substances determine brown sugar's 'super-calorie' qualities.

For the above experiments sugar comprised 90% of the calorie value of the rats' diet. The two following series of experiments took place under even harsher conditions of alimentary stress — the rats' food consisted only of white sugar or of brown sugar in equivalent amounts of sucrose. It was found that the two-month-old rats lived on almost identically for a further 30 days in both groups. In a similar experiment using 30-day-old rats a small and statistically insignificant difference was registered in brown sugar's favour. Therefore a comparison between the effects of white (sucrose) and brown sugar was carried out utilizing a wide range of dosages, from 0.5 g/kg to the total replacement of an entire feed by one sugar. In nearly all cases brown sugar in one way or another had several advantages over white sugar (sucrose).

Many facts are given in Yudkin's book in support of his claims that white sugar causes earlier maturation, increased growth and the appearance of illnesses which lead to diminished life span.[26] He also gives the results of some experiments on rats. In one of his experiments half the rats received sugar from the age of one month. Eight out of the 14 rats given a diet without sugar were still alive after two years, whereas only three out of the 14 in the experimental group had survived.

Then Yudkin reproduces the results of observations made by Dutch research workers who fed some rats in a control group with a mixture of foods representing the average Dutch diet, supplying about 15.5% of their calories with sugar. These male rats survived an average of 566 days (approximately 19 months).[68] When double the amount of sugar was fed the average life span of the male rats was reduced to 486 days (16 months). In the groups of female rats the life span was 607 days for the experimental and 582 for the control group. Translating these findings into human terms, Yudkin reckons that the consumption of extra white sugar could reduce people's lives by ten years or more. It is very hard to be convinced that these calculations are well-founded, but in their own right these experimental findings, despite their paucity, compel one to pay most serious attention to this aspect of white sugar's harmful effects.

All our findings about brown sugar's good points, the details of which are presented in this book, have made probable the suggestion that brown sugar, even in large doses, will shorten the life span of animals to a considerably lesser extent than white sugar will. But only by experiment can we be certain that this is the case.

For the following experiments we joined forces with Professor A.A. Meshcherskaya, who holds the chair of pharmacology at the Vladivostok Medical Institute. All in all the experiments were carried out using nearly 1,000 rats of both sexes. Starting when the animals were about 40 days old, the rats in the experimental groups were given throughout their lives a diet in which sucrose or brown sugar were substituted for 15%, 30% or 50% of the food's calorie value. These quantities correspond to 15 g/kg, 30 g/kg or 50 g/kg of sugar. The rats in the control group received their normal diet.

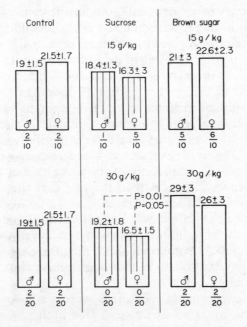

Figure 3. The influence of sucrose and brown sugar in amounts of 15 and 30 g/kg (15–30% of the diet calorie value) on the average life span of male and female rats in months.
Below the columns: the numerator denotes the number of rats in a group, and the denominator the number of rats living more than 30 months.

As can be seen from the findings in Figure 3, sucrose in a dose of 15 g/kg barely shortened the average life span of the male rats but noticeably reduced that of the female rats. By contrast, brown sugar in an equal dose prolonged average survival, even when compared with the control groups. The average life span was calculated for all the rats dying before two years were up. Of those which lived for more than 30 months, four rats were in the control group, six were fed on sucrose and 11 on brown sugar.

Even clearer results were obtained with a dose of sugars comprising 30% of the calorie value of the rats' diet (the lower group of columns in Figure 3). Sucrose had almost the same effect as when its dose was halved. But brown sugar had an even better effect: the male rats lived an average 29 ± 3.0 months and the females 26 ± 3.0 months (in both cases the difference when compared with sucrose is statistically significant). Not one rat on white sugar lived longer than 30 months, whereas 4 out of 40 rats did so on brown sugar.

In another series of experiments, rats in the control group received their normal, full-value food, while rats in the second and third groups had half their calories replaced by sucrose or brown sugar in a dose of approximately 50 g/kg. The weight gain of rats on both sugar regimens was reduced after three months compared with controls (control: 145 ± 6 g; sucrose: 125 ± 8 g). After 12 months of the experiment there was virtually no difference in the weight of rats in the three groups, but after two years, by which time rats in the control group weighed 306 ± 30 g, rats that had been eating brown sugar weighed somewhat less (244 ± 20 g) than those fed on sucrose (285 ± 25 g). K.A. Meshcherskaya is inclined to attribute the smaller weight increase of rats in the brown sugar group to the fact that they did not eat up all their daily food with brown sugar in it.

Observations of the general condition, behaviour and motor activity showed that in the first month brown sugar reduced the latent period of conditional reflex,[69] somewhat shortening the time, compared with sucrose, that the rats took to run through a maze, but afterwards this difference gradually levelled out.

In the same experiments recordings were made for 18 months of the liquids drunk by rats when given a free choice between water and 0.55% solutions of sucrose and brown sugar. It was demonstrated that prolonged consumption of brown sugar by rats significantly reduces sucrose consumption, which is definitely a positive result.

Of even greater importance are the findings about rats' preference for water or 20% alcohol when given the choice.[70] 20—40% of rats on a normal diet showed a preference for alcohol; white sugar increased this indicator to 40—60%, whereas brown sugar did not change it.

The effects of sucrose and brown sugar on the weight of certain organs was taken into account in the experiments that have been described. Thus after three months the thymus from rats which had been fed on brown or white sugar weighed less than the thymus from the controls, and by approximately the same amounts; after five months this difference was even more marked in rats that had been fed sucrose, but after nine months the weight of the thymus in the control was lower relatively, while in rats on both kinds of sugar it had returned close to its initial weight. Brown sugar, to a somewhat greater extent than sucrose, increased the average weight of the rats' ovaries and uterus, as was observed throughout two years. After 12 months brown sugar increased the average weight of the rats' testicles, prostate gland, and the regional anabolic muscle (*levator ani*) somewhat more than sucrose.

The divergence in the effects of sucrose and brown sugar had a detectable overall effect on the 15 rats belonging to each group. As the findings indicate (Table 5), a large total dose of brown sugar did not increase the rats' life span when compared with controls, but it did reduce it to a somewhat smaller extent than white sugar.

Table 5. The influence of sucrose and brown sugar (50 g/kg) on rats' life span

Conditions of the experiment	Death of the rats		Cause of death	Average life span, in months	Survived for over 24 months
	First incidence of death, in months				
Control	15	11	pneumonia	18.0 ± 2.0	7
Sucrose	15	7	necrotic tumours	15.0 ± 2.0	5
Brown sugar	15	8	pneumonia	16.2 ± 1.5	4

Pathohistological research has revealed that protracted dosage with sucrose induces diffuse cardiosclerosis and leads to fatty and granular degeneration of the liver in rats. When analogous amounts of brown sugar were taken by the rats these changes were less marked.

In this and previous chapters we have described the results of research, some already published, the chief aim of which has been to compare white with brown sugar in doses capable of producing an unfavourable effect on animals. With this end in view both kinds of sugar were fed in the majority of experiments to animals in amounts (30–50 g/kg), comprising 30–50% of the food calorie value. This level of sugar in the food was selected deliberately. In several developed countries the consumption of refined carbohydrates (sugar and white flour products) reaches precisely this level. The sugars were fed to the animals for many months and in several cases throughout their entire lives. Hence the experiments on the animals closely approximated to a dietary pattern widespread in western industrialized nations. We had not reckoned on obtaining any confirmation of specially positive aspects of brown sugar's action. Our chief objective has been to clarify whether, because of the natural additives it contains, brown sugar is less toxic than white. The results have surpassed our expectations. Brown sugar, even in a dose of 50 g/kg, is not only less toxic than white but has also shown itself to be a product that contributes to health.

Brown sugar causes animals to gain less weight than white; it increases their mobility and somewhat improves the state of the central nervous system. Both kinds of sugar have a slightly gonadotropic action but this has proved a positive factor with regard to the animal's reproductive function. To a greater extent than white, brown sugar shortens the mating period of female rats and the time till the first births, increasing the numbers of rats in the litters and their average weight, both in the first and second generations. Further research will enable a conclusive assessment to be made of all these effects of brown sugar's action on animals' reproductive functions. But even at the present stage it is clear that on this level brown sugar, even in large amounts, is no more dangerous than white. On the contrary, the gonadotropic action of brown sugar — or rather molasses — may find special application in certain areas of livestock breeding.

Rats who have eaten brown sugar are more resistant to stress induced by physical means (hanging) and alimentary stress (sugar loading of up to 90% of the food's calorie value).[70] Even when single and relatively small doses (1.0–2.2 g/kg) of brown sugar are given to white mice they elicit a definite increase in the animals' work capacity, an effect completely lacking in the action of white sugar.

The sum total of brown sugar's positive effects led to an increase in the rats' average life span, both in comparison with white sugar and with the control in which rats ate no sugar. For instance, female rats eating 30 g/kg of brown sugar lived on average 29 months, which is ten months longer than female rats on ordinary food. The difference for the male rats was only 4.5 months. On the basis that one month of a rat's life is equal to 2–3 years of a person's life, the difference represents an extra 9–30 years of human life expectancy. This calculation is purely hypothetical, it only serves to underline the magnitude of the difference in the length of the rats' lives.

Thus the complex of biologically active substances accompanying brown sugar make it not only a less harmful but, in many respects, a positively valuable product. The next chapter corroborates this conclusion with the results of studying the effect of white and brown sugar on certain categories of metabolism.

CHAPTER 8

The Influence of White and Brown Sugar on Metabolism

In Chapter 3 there was a short review of the pathology caused by excess consumption of refined carbohydrates, particularly white sugar. A leading position is held among these pathological shifts by illnesses caused by profound changes in metabolism.

Diabetes acquired with age has long been called confectioners' disease. The number of confections as such has not greatly increased, but the number of people ill with diabetes has gone on rising, a situation which has been directly linked in the recent decade with extra sugar consumption. Animal experiments have confirmed this. It has been found that the substitution of sucrose for 40–70% of rats' food calorie values reduces their sugar tolerance, which is followed by the manifestation of diabetes mellitus.[72] It is interesting to note that the frequency of diabetic illness in town dogs is four times higher than for dogs living in the country, receiving less carbohydrates in their food. Diabetes is also encountered in cats in towns, but the frequency is five times less than it is for dogs, presumably because cats eat far less sugar and confectionery.[73]

The beginning of the 1970s saw the accumulation of information from experiments showing that an increased carbohydrate content (40–70% of the calorie value) of rats' food accelerates the synthesis of fatty acids, the structural lipids, cholesterol and other metabolites implicated in disturbances of lipid metabolism. Then it was established that the pattern of disturbance of lipid metabolism is intensified when there is a deficiency of protein intake.[74] Investigations into the changes in lipid metabolism provoked by sucrose revealed retardation of lipolysis and oxidation of fatty acids, reduced activity of glucose-6-phosphates[75] and many other alterations.

Literature relating to research and clinical observations concerned with the action of refined carbohydrates on carbohydrate and lipid metabolism is extremely extensive and is contradictory on several points. Nevertheless the vast majority of workers agree that the oligosaccharides and di-saccharides, particularly sucrose, are the chief culprits of the pathological shifts occurring in metabolism. It has been noticed that refined starch and natural foodstuffs containing starch do not have the same effects — indeed, they often lower the blood cholesterol level; moreover, the greater the amount of natural substances (cellulose, vegetable fibre, pectin) in a foodstuff, the more they promote the excretion of cholesterol from the body.[76]

Despite the large number of works on the harmful effects of brown sugar, most of them are concerned with individual and rather narrow aspects of metabolism. The majority of the experiments are limited to a few weeks, occasionally to a few months. It is very seldom that the items being investigated are any substances or products which could be regarded as potential antagonists of white sugar. However strange it may appear, the fact remains that brown sugar has almost never been studied in parallel with white sugar.

The present chapter presents the results of many years of joint research with Professor K.A. Meshcherskaya and her colleagues at the chair of Pharmacology Unit, Vladivostok Medical Institute.

Over 720 Wistar (mongrel) rats were used in this work. Different series of animals were given chemically pure sucrose or brown sugar in differing amounts: 2 g/kg, 15 g/kg or 50 g/kg, representing from 2—50% of their daily food intake in calories. Brown sugar was given in slightly bigger amounts (to correct for the percentage content of the nonsaccharides) in order to balance the amount of sucrose that both groups of animals received. Various sets of observations were made at 15-day intervals and then after 3, 5, 9, 12 months and longer. The research encompassed a broad spectrum of indicators of carbohydrate and protein metabolism, with histological examination of certain organs completing the projects.

We focus here on the results of the 3-month experiments, for which there is fuller data that lends itself to better comparison. Figure 4 (see also ref. 77 — Table) illustrates the steady increase in the blood sugar level that accompanies increased intake of white sugar. However, approximately the same amounts of brown sugar do not cause a noticeable increase in the rats' blood sugar level, even in a dose of 50 g/kg, which amounts to half the calorie value of their daily food. After five months the elevated blood sugar level of rats receiving white sugar in this large dose was maintained, and only returned to normal after nine months, a response which may be regarded as the first sign of physiological adaptation to the high amount of sugar being consumed. In rats on an equally high dose of brown sugar virtually the first indication of physiological adaptation to sugar came towards the end of the third month, i.e. 6 months earlier.

A similar picture emerges from the quantitative indicators of the changes in liver and muscle glycogen content, except that the muscle glycogen of rats receiving the large dose of brown sugar was markedly increased.

Brown sugar caused a smaller change in blood and liver indicators of lipid metabolism than sucrose (Figure 5, see also Table, ref. 78). Of significance were the results of Cuncel's test, which indicated an impairment of serum protein binding ability with cholesterol. As shown in Figure 6 brown sugar fared better than white in this test as well.

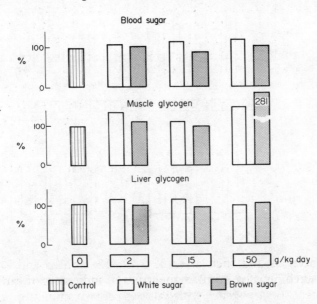

Figure 4. The influence of different quantities of sucrose and brown sugar on certain indicators of carbohydrate metabolism in rats.

Histological examination verified that prolonged consumption by rats of sucrose leads to changes in the myocardium of the diffuse cardiosclerotic type, with fatty and granulated atrophy detected in the liver. Brown sugar triggered less marked changes in these organs.

Because people take sugar throughout their lives it was important to determine its effect on the blood coagulating system, since any findings could be of particular significance with regard to middle-aged and older people. This research was undertaken at the Pharmacology Unit of the Medical Faculty of the Patrice Lumumba University of People's Friendship in Moscow by Prof. S.I. Zolotukhin and Drs. V.F. Kremneva, A.I. Pozharska and T.S. Sorokina. The experiments were carried out on 200 rats and 150 rabbits into whose stomachs sucrose or brown sugar was fed in daily doses of 2 g/kg or 15 g/kg for 30, 60 or

90 days. The animals in the control group were dosed with an isotonic solution of sodium chloride. It was established that both sucrose and brown sugar in a 15 g/kg daily dose shorten the blood coagulation time, heighten the animals' sensitivity to heparin, and activate the anticoagulating system. No difference was detected between the action of sucrose and that of brown sugar.

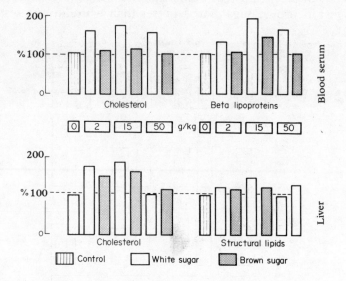

Figure 5. The influence of different amounts of sucrose and brown sugar on certain indicators of lipid metabolism in rats.

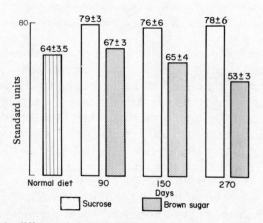

Figure 6. The difference in indicators of the Cuncel (unit) test in the prolonged feeding of rats (50 g/kg) daily on sucrose or brown sugar.

In conclusion, then, the results of the research described in this chapter demonstrate that white sugar causes serious disturbances in carbohydrate and lipid metabolism. These findings are in agreement with those of other writers. Brown sugar in equal amounts to sucrose causes substantially less metabolic disturbance, which may be regarded as a very important contribution to our total knowledge of brown sugar's valuable effects.

CHAPTER 9

Sugar and Dental Caries

Mammals have the same teeth as man, but in the wild they never have dental caries. Caries is a purely human acquisition. But why should man have inflicted this misery upon himself? There is one thing that scientists are in agreement about, and this is concerning the role of carbohydrates, and especially refined white sugar, in the development of caries. It is sucrose that is responsible for caries. By means of a saliva invertase, sucrose splits into glucose and fructose, with the subsequent formation of lactic acid, an energy-rich substance that promotes the development of the *Streptococcus mutans* microbe. Streptococcus, in its turn, intervenes in the sugar division process, resulting in the formation of the intermediary product dextrin. Dextrin does not dissolve in water but forms plaque ('tartar') that adheres to the teeth. Vast numbers of microbes, which secrete acid, form in the plaque, destroying the dentine. Hence the following are important in prophylaxis: a) strengthening the dentine; b) removal of plaque (cleaning teeth and removing encrustations); c) reducing sugar intake.

It must not be thought that modern man's dentine differs greatly from the dentine of his ancestors or of wild animals. Dentine's lowered resistance to caries arises because of a deficiency of certain trace elements, fluorine in particular, that occur only in limited areas. It cannot be said that people in developed countries do not clean their teeth. And yet it is precisely the population of these countries that are affected by caries. The Eskimos of Alaska, the bushmen and Bantu races in Africa, and also the aborigines on certain islands, with virtually no contact with the civilized world, practically never suffer from dental caries. But when contact with Europeans has been extended and the nature of their food has changed, with refined carbohydrates and especially white sugar appearing in it, caries has affected them in increasingly large numbers. There is no doubt that caries is an ecological problem.[79]

R.H. Hall has produced some interesting facts about caries in Greeks, the French, Danes and the British during a period of 5,000 years, from Neolithic man to the present day.[19] For more than 4,500 years the percentage of people with dental caries seldom exceeded 4—8% and it is only in the last two to three centuries that it has risen to 24%.

It is perfectly obvious that it is not a matter of the quantity of sugar eaten but of how it enters the body. G.D. Campbell has shown that sugar-cane cutters in South Africa eat certain parts of the plant in amounts containing 400 g of sugar.[80] But despite the fact that on mastication 79—83% of the sugar total is drawn out into the person's mouth, it was found that these cutters were almost entirely free from caries. Another research investigation revealed that it was sufficient to wash the oral cavity of healthy people with a sucrose solution nine times daily over a fortnight, for changes to be induced in the teeth resembling the early stages of caries.[81] The same group of authors established that the demineralization of dental enamel that takes place during rinsing was not reduced by the addition of 1% calcium glycerophosphate to the sucrose solution, but its growth was retarded by the local application of a 2% solution of sodium fluoride.[82]

The addition of sodium fluoride to drinking water has been the only measure against caries to have received more or less widespread implementation. Food additives such as non-organic and organic phosphates, vitamin D, vitamin B_6, molybdenum, vanadium and other trace elements, antioxidants, complexing agents and other substances have proved less effective.[83]

Like a drop of water, the particular problem of sugar's role in spreading caries reflects in itself all the aspects of the overall problem of sugar! As often as not the measures ranged against caries also turn out to be ineffective or difficult to implement. More than 40 years ago T.W.B. Osborn and his co-workers postulated the hypothesis that certain kinds of food contain a protective factor against caries.[84] As for the carbohydrates, the main culprits of caries, they also are accompanied in nature by a 'protective agent', which to a greater or lesser extent is removed during the refining process. This has been repeatedly confirmed *in vitro* and on laboratory animals while examining several natural foods, including wheat grain (ground and in extract form) and whole cocoa powder, among others.[85]

Of special interest in this connection is A. Strålfors's research project on golden hamsters which received either a normal diet or one to which white (control) or brown sugar had been added. Molasses was the supplement in one of his experiments. Table 6, which is derived from his 1966 paper, shows that brown sugar and molasses caused a greater increase in the weight of the hamsters and 68—78% less dental caries than white sugar.

Table 6. The effect of brown sugar and molasses on the weight of golden hamsters
and on caries in a 45-day experiment (A. Strålfors, 1966)

Experiment	Conditions of the experiment	Amount of sugar, %	Increased body weight, g	Reduced dental caries, %
A	White sugar, powder	50	28.4	
	Brown sugar, crystals	50	41.3	68
B	White sugar, solution	40	23.3	
	Brown sugar, solution	40	52.7	70
C	Sucrose	10		
	Glucose	5	37.9	
	Fructose	5		
	Molasses	20	56.8	78

Table 7. The incidence of dental caries in rats fed for 60 days on a cariogenic diet
of white or brown sugar compared with rats fed their usual diet

Diet	Number of rats	Average weight at end of experiment, g	Average number of dental caries per rat	Average amount of cariogenic damage per rat
Normal diet	37	92.5 ± 5.6	1.0 ± 0.1	1.1 ± 0.1
Cariogenic diet with white sugar	20	59.6 ± 3.6	9.2 ± 0.3 $p = 0.001$	13.7 ± 0.04 $p = 0.01$
Cariogenic diet with brown sugar	21	92.6 ± 5.4	5.8 ± 0.4 $p = 0.001$	6.7 ± 0.08 $p = 0.001$

Strålfors's findings were confirmed by an experimental research group of the Odessa Medical Institute (I.M. Dmitriyev, A.G. Zalogina, N.V. Kaliberdina, R.F. Makulkin, Yu.A. Fedorov, G.V. Filin and A.A. Shandra). The experiments were carried out on 30-day-old Wistar rats fed a cariogenic diet for 60 days: casein — 18%; dried crusts — 18%; sunflower oil — 5%; saline mixture — 4% (sodium chloride — 100 g; calcium chloride — 3 g; potassium chloride — 0.5 g; mono-calcium phosphate — 0.5 g; calcium sulphate — 0.5 g; pulverized sulphur — 0.1 g; the salts of zinc sulphate, copper, cobalt, and ferrous chloride in traces); and 54% of either white or brown sugar. As Table 7 indicates, the cariogenic diet containing white sugar substantially retarded the animals' development and sharply increased the incidence of dental caries. Brown sugar in the same cariogenic diet did not retard development and the incidence of dental caries was approximately half that caused by white sugar. Brown sugar had a slight prophylactic effect against periodonitis.

Electrocardiographic and electroencephalographic readings of the rats fed the cariogenic diet revealed changes characteristic of experimental atherosclerosis. These changes were significantly less marked in rats fed the diet containing brown sugar. Morphological examination highlighted the changes conditioned by sugar loading, which represented a similar picture to diabetes mellitus. In rats fed the diet containing brown sugar these changes began later and were less pronounced.

Radiological estimations of sulphur-32 and phosphorus-32 accumulated in rat tissues showed that brown sugar had a less marked effect on protein and mineral metabolism than white sugar. Spectrographic emission indicated that brown sugar's prophylactic action against dental caries might also be explained by it in some way preserving the relative stability of the trace element content in dental tissues.

Finally, those who participated in this research project reached the conclusion that the partial substitution of brown for white sugar could have an important role in prophylactic measures designed to combat human dental caries.

CHAPTER 10

The Effects of Brown Sugar on Man: Some Observations

The total findings from experiments on laboratory animals show that brown sugar lacks nearly all white sugar's shortcomings and, moreover, that it is without doubt a valuable dietary product for animals. Nevertheless objective accounts of its effects on people must provide the last word, since we are the ones for whom brown sugar is intended. Research into a new medicine or food product follows the two main aims of establishing their harmlessness and determining their useful qualities. Life itself represents an almost global experiment in the use of brown sugar. In this no suspicion has ever been attached to brown sugar's toxicity. Mention has been made in previous chapters of certain epidemiological statistics, according to which the consumption of brown sugar by the population of several countries has been linked with the lower incidence of cardiovascular diseases or caries. But this evidence can only be regarded as indirect evidence of brown sugar's value. We have not been able to find any written work describing brown sugar's valuable effects on people.

V.Sh. Belkin and A.L. Vovsi-Kolshteyn, researchers at the Tadzhik SSR Academy of Science's Mountain Medico-Biological Research Laboratory, carried out the first project. Under observation were two groups of healthy young men of approximately the same age, who had just arrived in a mountainous area 3,600 metres above sea-level where they were confronted by the difficulties of both adapting to the altitude and working over a long period. In the experimental group brown sugar replaced 20 g of sugar. In the control group all the sugar eaten was refined. Research was conducted in accordance with the double-blind method. Before the start of observations, again after a month, and then at three-monthly intervals, several subjective indicators were examined (complaints, sleep, appetite, fatiguability and others), as well as objective ones (frequency of consulting a doctor, incidence of catarrhal illnesses, body weight, pulse beat, arterial pressure, and blood picture, including particulars of general blood analysis and the amount of protein and sugar present).

People usually voice many different complaints during the first days and weeks of living at high altitude. The most frequent complaints of the young men in this study were headaches, giddiness, dyspnoea tachycardia, reduced appetite, somnolence, debility, difficulty in falling asleep, irritability and so forth. As may be seen from the tabulated results,[87] during the first month of living under mountainous conditions members of the control (white sugar) group complained more often for adaptation reasons than the brown sugar group. The data obtained indicates that brown sugar facilitates the more rapid and effective development of the compensatory mechanisms of the adaptation process. During the subsequent months the number of complaints continued to fall but the differences between the groups evened out to some extent in the course of a year.

Body weight is an objective indicator of the process of adaptation. The first weeks of high-altitude living usually see a loss of weight and then its gradual recovery (Figure 7). In the control group the initial

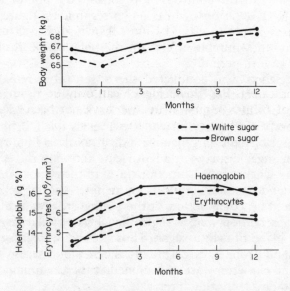

Figure 7. Brown sugar's influence on body weight and the red blood indicators
of young people adapting to mountainous conditions (see findings of
V.Sh. Belkin and A.L. Vovsi-Kolshteyn).

body weight fell by over 1 kg during the first month; then recovery of the lost weight started, but by the end of the year there was still a difference between the average body weight of those on white and those on brown sugar. During the initial and most arduous adaptation period the average weight of the men in the group on brown sugar fell by only 300 g, while the initial weight of those tested was regained one month ahead of the control group.

The dynamics of adaptative changes in pulse frequency and arterial pressure at rest was roughly identical in both groups, but in the first month, with medicated physical overloads, the time required for the pulse rate and arterial pressure level to return to normal values was reduced by 15—20% under the influence of brown sugar. From the findings presented in Figure 7 it is clear that a change in the red cell parameters (erythrocyte count and haemoglobin content) testifies to the greater activity of the adaptation processes in people taking brown sugar. In this study brown sugar promoted the development of adaptive compensatory mechanisms. During the first weeks brown sugar caused somewhat less of a fall in the blood sugar level, and the serum protein and blood serum content of both groups under test conditions was virtually the same. During the year spent in mountainous conditions members of the control group consulted a doctor about various illnesses on 41 occasions, while the corresponding figure for those in the brown sugar group was 31 times. Brown sugar was not discovered to have any unfavourable effects on the people who took it throughout the 12-month period.

The specialists who conducted the observations remarked in their report on the fact that brown sugar has the ability to secure better coordination of the compensatory mechanisms, especially during the initial period of adaptation, which expresses itself in improved subjective sensations and in objective indicators. It is important to stress that brown sugar displays its adaptogenic action in the early period of adaptation, when bodily functions are at their most unstable level.

The second research project on people was organized by V.A. Shibanov and his collaborators at the Vladivostok Medical Institute.

Under observation were 237 people who every day received 70 g of brown in place of white sugar. Those tested were observed various times, ranging from 37 to 218 days. Their blood serum sugar, β-lipoproteins and cholesterol were examined at the beginning of the experiment and then at monthly intervals.

Table 8 gives the data for the effect of brown sugar, taken for approximately four months, on a group of people in whom the initial indicators of carbohydrate and lipid metabolism were elevated. In these people all three biochemical indicators of the metabolic state were substantially returned to normal values. For the entire period that brown sugar was taken, and for several months afterwards, no

Table 8. The influence of the prolonged (110–122 days) consumption of
brown sugar on certain blood serum biochemical indicators

Indicators	Units of measurement	Number of people	Before	After
Sugar	mg %	25	145 ± 6.0	109 ± 4.5 p < 0.0001
β-lipoproteins	units	20	52 ± 2.0	27 ± 1.4 p < 0.0001
Cholesterol	mg %	30	299 ± 7.8	190 ± 3.0 p < 0.0001

negative phenomena were noticed. Against the background of normal blood sugar, cholesterol and β-lipoprotein indicators, no changes occurred in their levels. There was not a special control group in this experiment, but those who obtained brown sugar in certain dishes were not aware of the fact.

Thus brown sugar has had a favourable effect upon people in ordinary life and under conditions of stress.

Conclusions

The material that has been presented are the results of comprehensive and, one might say, rigorous tests designed to compare the effects of white and brown sugar. The tests were rigorous because the animals received diets consisting of 50–90% sugar, and the experiments were continued for several months, sometimes for an animal's life-time. Factors considered included the development of young and adult animals, the state of the reproductive functions, effects on the foetus and on the development of new-born offspring, resistance to the effects of stress, work endurance to the point of complete exhaustion, various indicators of carbohydrate and lipid metabolism, the condition of the teeth, and the length of the animals' lives.

As one might have expected, white sugar revealed all its negative aspects. All the data obtained, the main items of which have been summarized under Table 9, prove that white sugar lowers the 'vital potential' of animals' bodies. They become less able to resist stress, their reproductive functions become less efficient, their metabolism is impaired, the incidence of dental caries increases, and several other adverse changes have been observed. The conclusion from this is that white sugar, when taken in amounts closely approximating those usually consumed by people, leads to premature ageing. We saw this for ourselves, *ad oculus*, during prolonged observation of the animals. Compared with the controls, rats which ate white sugar were less clean and mobile, showed less interest in the opposite sex, and lost their reproductive functions at an earlier stage. As a result these rats' average life span, as demonstrated by several experiments, was 13–17% shorter than the average life span of the controls. It should be emphasized that in research into brown sugar's anti-lipidaemic action there was no need to resort to any kind of model of experimental atherosclerosis as white sugar itself provoked a fairly serious picture of disturbances of lipid metabolism. The same could be said of changes in carbohydrate metabolism, which were quite grave when caused by white sugar.

Table 9. Some data comparing the effects of white and brown sugar on animals

Indicators		White sugar	Brown sugar
The increase in work time of mice to complete exhaustion in stimulating units of action (SUA in 1 g)		0	25–55
Stress resistance		lowered	raised
Trophic value cumulative indicator		0.77	1.01
Changes in the blood's biochemical indicators as percentages of control (50% food's calorie value sugar — for 90 days)	Sugar	124	105
	Cholesterol	149	103
	β-lipoproteins	164	100
Overall embryonic foetal loss as percentage of control (90% food's calorie value sugar — for 20 days)		175	69
An increase compared with control of the average number of dental caries per rat (54% food's calorie value sugar — for 60 days)		12 times	6 times
Change in rats' average life span as percentage of control (30% food's calorie value sugar — for lifetime)		87% (17.8 months)	134% (25.5 months)

In experiments conducted in parallel with brown sugar the animals obtained the same amount of sucrose as that contained in the administered dose of white sugar. But it requires only 4% of the substances accompanying sucrose in brown sugar to radically alter the picture. First and foremost any apprehension that we might have felt that brown sugar was toxic or dangerous on account of certain impurities in it were rapidly dispelled. On the contrary, it proved to be considerably less harmful than white sugar. Indeed only one experimental fact is needed to back up this statement — white sugar, in comparison with control, increases the average number of carious teeth by a factor of 12, brown sugar by a factor of only 6. All the remaining information (see, for instance, Table 9) is proof that brown sugar, in contradistinction to white sugar, is a valuable product. It increases animals' work capacity and resistance to stress, almost entirely eliminates evidence of white sugar's harmful effects on carbohydrate and lipid metabolism, and reduces embryo loss to below the level of that of the control animals. In a series of experiments the average life span of rats receiving brown sugar all their lives turned out to be higher than a similar indicator for the control group of rats which received an ordinary diet without sugar.

For the last ten years we have struggled to answer the question often put to us: 'What is better, to give up sugar altogether or to eat brown sugar?' Now, on the basis of the sum total of our findings we can reply that it is best to eat brown sugar. This kind of sugar retains all sucrose's nutritious and palatable qualities (it is even tastier than white sugar), and it not only lacks the latter's harmful effects but has valuable properties that actually promote health. Perhaps our reply is too categorical, and for a definitive answer what is needed is more extensive data from human studies than we have described in the last chapter. But so far all our results point in favour of brown sugar. In confirmation of this one may adduce to a certain extent epidemiological findings about the reduced susceptibility of people to atherosclerosis and cardiovascular illnesses in countries where unrefined sugars are used. However, the living conditions of people in these countries are distinguished not merely by the purity of sugar but by a host of other things as well. It is difficult, though in principle possible (and necessary), to carry out observations in several towns varying in size, half the population of which is to receive only white sugar for several years, while the other half receives only brown sugar. There are grounds for believing that after some years it would be possible to detect a difference in the overall illness rate, in the frequency of atherosclerosis and cardiovascular diseases, and in dental caries. Were observations of this kind to be extended for several decades it is possible that the average life span might also have lengthened. There is no doubt whatsoever that factors in food are infinitely superior to medicines for prolonging life — medicines sought, but never found by striving scientists. Even when and if reliably effective medicines are discovered for making life longer it will hardly be everyone that uses them. For many people they will remain medicines towards which their attitudes will be contradictory. Even when a person is ill he often feels an inner resistance to taking medicines, often regarding them as an inevitable ill or evil, given a specific situation. However, when a person thinks he is well this inner resistance becomes immeasurably greater. It is no small matter to decide at what age one begins to take medicines to increase life expectancy. So far there is no answer to this question because there are no such medicines. But when they do appear it will be very difficult to find the right answer to this question.

One can anticipate that objections will be raised at our assertions about the non-existence of geriatric pharmacological medicines on the grounds that they are too categorical. It is true that this science has proposed complexes of vitamins and anti-oxidants. But leaving aside synthetic preparations with an anti-oxidant action, even vitamins have not been used that widely by healthy people with the object of achieving such a living goal as increasing their span of active life. There are many reasons for this. There are so many different variants of vitamin complexes that it is open to question whether scientists and doctors really know what quantity, and in what combination, vitamins should be recommended for people of different ages. Moreover, there is a suspicion that vitamins dispensed from a chemist's shelf are not so effective as when they come from natural vegetable and animal products. Would it not be better to obtain the vitamins, the same anti-oxidants and the many other biologically active substances necessary to a person in the form of a complex of natural foodstuffs created by Nature herself? Then all the psychological barriers erected by man faced with medicines from useful biologically active substances would also disappear.

The entire complex of brown sugar's useful biologically active substances, that is, virtually any given section of molasses, could be made into beautiful little tablets to be carried in a packet in the pocket. But is it not better simply to eat brown sugar? Certainly. And from what age? All through life, is the answer. Ultimately the problem of active longevity can be solved only in the context of the solution of the more universal problem of the health of healthy people. And conditioning health should commence not merely with childhood or even infancy but inside the womb.

As may be seen from the results we have obtained, brown sugar ensures the birth of healthier and more vigorous progeny. In addition to the findings given in Table 4 and Figure 1, we would like to describe some observations which we have not managed to provide in figures. When female rats were autopsied on the eve of giving birth it was discovered that there was a clearly-marked difference in the foetuses. Living and moving foetuses were found in the wombs of rats which had received throughout gestation their usual food or brown sugar forming 90% of their calorie intake. But in rats fed the same amount of white sugar it was only possible to tell if a foetus was alive or dead by touching it. White sugar led to wrinkled, cyanotic foetuses with porous tissue which lacerated under pincers. Under the influence of white sugar the rat foetuses had already aged at the uterine stage; this did not happen with brown sugar.

Great is the force of habit, and brown sugar is not to everyone's liking. However, there will always be a choice since it is hard to imagine that white sugar will ever fall completely out of use. There is reason to hope that in time the adherents of white sugar will dwindle away and the sugar industry will have to change over to making brown sugar more than half of their production output. In nearly all cases brown sugar could be used for the so-called invisible sugar in confectionery goods, sweets, chocolates, condensed milk, soft drinks, ice-cream, beer, wines and other products. Both white and brown sugar chocolates and various confectionery items were made simultaneously at the chair of the Manufacture of Foodstuffs at the Far East Technical Institute for the Fishing Industry under the direction of S.B. Golikova. The members of the tasting commission were unable to discern what food contained which sugar, and on the whole the same assessments were made for both sugars. The specialists noticed that in several of the technological processes, brown sugar behaves differently from white but that it is easy to adapt to some of brown sugar's characteristics. Sometimes brown sugar imparts to products a pleasant taste and longer preservative qualities.

We hope that the time will not be far off when brown as opposed to white sugar will be given the widest preferential distribution. When taken over many years brown sugar will definitely be good for people's health. But in addition to resolving this great and important practical problem research into brown sugar has very real scientific significance.

The first task of this research is to obtain experimental confirmation of the importance of preserving the natural complex of the biologically active substances in food products, and corroborating the value of a defined quantity of structural information. As yet we still have not been able to calculate (in bits) the quantity of structural information of the approximately 200 organic compounds (of course there are many more) contained in the natural complex of brown sugar's substances. But there is no doubt that the amount is many times greater than the structural information present in a molecule of sucrose. Who knows, perhaps in the not too distant future two labels will appear on different sorts of sugar and on all other foodstuffs: one with the number of calories, the other with the amount of structural information.

The second important feature of the use of brown instead of white sugar on a world-wide scale would be the first case of scientifically substantiated production — neogathering (see Chapter 2) — whereby all the wealth and health of natural biologically active substances would be available to everyone without the family or the individual being put to any extra trouble or expense. In the first chapter we wrote about the importance of developing a doctrine about the psychology of health, because health depends to a very large extent on a person, on his or her awareness. But even when the elements of a psychology of health become common property it will be difficult for each person or family to be sure that they are taking the requisite optimum of biologically active substances (structural information) in their daily food. It will be the task of industrial neogathering to ensure that this happens.

Finally, a third aspect of the scientific significance of the results of brown sugar studies is that they accentuate the urgent need for similar research on other highly refined mass-consumer goods such as flour, vegetable oil and alcohol.

It was the genius of our remote ancestors that led them to find and cultivate cereals, oil and sugar-yielding plants and the grape vine. From them they made simple natural foods which, together with meat, formed the most important chemical factors in the progress and evolution of mankind.[88] But man armed with science and technology attempts to correct and improve nature, often only to find that the results are the reverse of what he expected.

The key to the health and long life of this and future generations lies in combining the millennial experience of our ancestors with the great possibilities of modern science and technology.

References and notes

1. G.T. Stewart (1975), 'Medicine and health: what connection?' *The Lancet,* 29 March, 706–708.
2. V.P. Kaznacheyev (1973), *The Biosystem and Adaptation.* Novosibirsk (R).
3. M. Sokolowska (1978), 'Medicine and society in the period of scientific and technical revolution', *Problemy,* 3, 12–20 (Polish).
4. J.S. Chapman (1974), 'Health and medicine', *Archives of Environmental Health,* 28 June, 350–351.
5. I.V. Davydovsky (1962), *Problems of Cause and Result in Medicine (Aetiology),* 'Meditsina', Moscow (R).
6. I.I. Brekhman (1976), *Man and Biologically Active Substances,* 'Nauka', Leningrad (R).
   I.I. Brekhman (1980), *Man and Biologically Active Substances: the Effect of Drugs, Diet and Pollution on Health,* Pergamon Press.
7. *The Principle of Complimentarity and Materialistic Dialectics,* 'Nauka', Moscow (1976) (R).
8. I.I. Brekhman (1957), *Ginseng,* Gosudarstvennoye izdatelstvo meditsinskoy literatury, Leningrad (R);
   I.I. Brekhman (1968), *Eleutherococcus,* 'Nauka', Leningrad (R);
   I.V. Dardymov (1976), *Ginseng and Eleutherococcus: Towards a Mechanism of Biological Activity,* 'Nauka', Moscow (R).
9. Hans Selye (1974), *Stress Without Distress,* McClelland and Stewart, Toronto.
10. I.I. Brekhman and I.F. Nesterenko (1971), 'The tranquillizing action of an extract of the saiga's horns', *Farmakologiya i toksikologiya,* 1, 36–38 (R).
11. L. Pauling (1971), *Vitamin C and the Common Cold,* Bantam Books.
12. D.D. Venediktov, A.M. Chernukh, Yu.P. Lisitsin and V.I. Krichagin (1979), 'Worldwide problems of health care and ways of solving them', *Voprosy filosofii,* 7, 102–113 (R).
13. A.A. Pokrovsky (1976), 'Food and illness', *Voprosy pitaniya,* 1, 18–33 (R).
14. K.H. Cooper (1970), *The New Aerobics,* M. Evans, New York.
15. V.V. Milashevich (1976), *The Methods and Fundamental Principles of Psychology,* Izdaniye Dalnevostochnogo gosudarstvennogo universiteta, Vladivostok (R).

16. W. Schoenenberger (1976), *Healthy Through Natural Juices. The Possibilities and Successes of Fresh Plants' Therapy*, Econ Verlag, Düsseldorf and Wien (G) (quoted in Russian translation, 'Znaniye').

17. A.A. Pokrovsky (1978), 'Food as the bearer and forerunner of biologically active substances', *Zhurnal Vsesoyuznogo khimicheskogo obshchestva im. D.I. Mendeleyeva*, **23**, 4, 363–371 (R).

18. Karl Marx and Friedrich Engels (1956), From their early *Works*, Gosudarstvennoye izdatelstvo politicheskoy literatury, Moscow, 564 (R).

19. R.H. Hall (1976), *Food for Nought. The Decline in Nutrition*, Vintage Books, New York.

20. R.H. Hall (1975), 'Is nutrition a stagnation science?' *New Scientist*, **62**, 970, 7–9.

21. L. Brillyuen (1966), *Scientific nonspecificity and information*, 'Mir', Moscow (R);
A.V. Katsura (1973), 'Informational aspects of the problem of the optimization of the biosphere', *The reciprocity of nature and society (philosophical, geographical, and ecological aspects of the problem)*, Moscow, 342–352 (R).

22. N. Viner (1968), *Cybernetics or Control and Communication in Animals and Machines*, 2nd edition, 'Sovetskoye radio', Moscow (R).

23. E. Shrödinger (1972), *What is life? From the Physics Viewpoint*, 2nd edition, 'Atomizdat', Moscow (R).

24. S.M. Dancoff and H. Quastler (1953), 'The information content and error rate of living things', in *Information theory in biology*. University of Illinois Press, Urbana, 263–273.

25. I.B. Novik (1974), 'Physics and the biosphere (methodological aspect)', in *The Future of Science. The Natural Sciences and Ecology*, Dubna, 5–8 (R).

26. J. Yudkin (1974), *Pure, White and Deadly. The Problem of Sugar*. Davis-Poynter.

27. A. Hoffer (1977), 'Supernutrition', in *A physician's Handbook on Orthomolecular Medicine*, edited by R.J. Williams and D.K. Kalita, Pergamon Press.

28. C. Loewenfeld (1978), *Everything you Should Know about your Food*, Faber and Faber.

29. E.P. Vagane (1976), *Some Nutrition and Metabolism Characteristics of the Estonian SSR Population*, 'Valgus', Tallinn (R).

30. P.E. Norris (1975), *About Molasses*, Thorsons Publishers, Wellingborough.

31. G.G. Birch, M. Spencer and A.G. Cameron (1977), *Food Science*, 2nd edition, Pergamon Press.

32. R.C. Atkins (1972), *Dr Atkins's Diet Revolution*, David McKay, New York.

33. S.G. Genes (1970), *Hypoglycaemia. The Hypoglycaemic Complex of Syndromes*, 'Meditsina', Moscow (R).
(S. Harris, in *The Journal of the American Medical Association*, **83**, (1924), 729–733, quoted by Genes).

34. R. Adams and F. Murray (1974), *Megavitamin Therapy*, Larchamont Books, New York; E. Cheraskin and W.M. Ringsdorf, Jun., with A. Brecher (1974), *Psychodietetics: Food as the Key to Emotional Health*, Steind and Day, New York; R. Adams and F. Murray (1975), *Is Low Blood Sugar Making you a Nutritional Cripple?* Larchamont Books, New York; R.C. Atkins (1975), 'Introduction', in the book: *Is Low Blood Sugar Making you a Nutritional Cripple?* Larchamont Books, New York; H. Ross (1975), *Fighting Depression*, Larchamont Books, New York; and W. Currier, J. Baron and D.K. Kalita (1977), 'The end of your sweet life', in *A Physician's Handbook on Ortho-molecular Medicine*, Pergamon Press, 156—160.

35. S.J. O'Keefe and V. Marks (1977), 'Lunchtime gin and tonic. A cause of reactive hypoglycaemia', *The Lancet*, **8025**, 1286—1288.

36. M. Damyanova, M. Atanasova, Tsv. Damyanova, L. Khristov, V. Petrova, A. Ilkov, and O. Koparanova (1978), 'Insulin secretion, glucose assimilation and the level of free fatty acids in children with adiposis', *Pediatriya*, **17**, 4, 361—366 (Bulgarian).

37. I.T. Kalyuzhny and V.D. Zharova (1977), 'Adiposis and diabetes mellitus', *Sb. nauchnykh trudov Kirgizskogo meditsinskogo instituta*, **123**, 82—87 (R).

38. C.N. Tobares, T. Diaz De La Pena, T. De Los Santos Baez, and L.F. Guillen (1978), 'The diabetic patient in geriatrics. A Comparative study between hospitalized and ambulatory patients', *Revista española gerontologia y geriatria*, **13**, 1, 47—58 (Spanish).

39. P. Zimmer, M. Arblastor and K. Thoma (1978), 'The effect of westernization on native populations. Studies on a Microneisan community with a high diabetes prevalence', *Australian and New Zealand Journal of Medicine*, **8**, 2, 141—146.

40. See, for instance, D. Greenstock (1977), 'Atherosclerosis and the refined carbohydrates', *Ecologist*, **7**, 9, 362—365; W. Lutz (1977), 'Nutrition and risk factors', *Wiener medizinische Wochenschrift*, **127**, 7, 222—225 (G); J. Yudkin (1978), 'Dietary factors in arteriosclerosis: sucrose', *Lipids*, **13**, 5, 370—372; and many others.

41. M.H. Robinson (1977), 'On sugar and white flour . . . the dangerous twins!' in *A Physician's Handbook on Orthomolecular Medicine*, Pergamon Press, 24—30.

42. P.M. Gaman and K.B. Sherington (1977), *The Science of Food. An Introduction to Food Science, Nutrition and Microbiology*, Pergamon Press.

43. K.J. Parker (1978), 'Alternatives to sugar. The search for an ideal non-nutritive sweetener is almost a century old', *Nature (London)*, **271**, 493—495.

44. See note 31.

45. B. Commoner (1971), *The Closing Circle. Nature, Man, Technology*, New York.

46. R. Adams and F. Murray (1974), *Minerals: Kill or Cure?* Larchamont Books, New York.

47. H.A. Schroeder (1974) 'The role of trace elements in cardiovascular disease', *Medical Clin. of North America*, **58**, 2, 381–396.
48. R.H. Davis, C.A. Albert, D.L. Kramer and J. Sackman (1974), 'Atherogenic effect of sucrose and white flour fed to obese mice, *Experientia*, **30**, 8, 910–911; and N.A. Worcester, K.B. Brucdorfer and J. Yudkin (1975), 'The effect of dietary sucrose and different dietary fats on hyperlipidemia and atherosclerosis on white Leghorn cockerels (*Gallus domesticus*)', *Proceedings of the Nutrition Society*, **34**, 2, 82–83.
49. P.B. Disler, S.R. Lynch, R.W. Charlton, T.H. Bothwell, R.B. Walker and F. Mayet (1975), 'Studies on the fortification of cane sugar with iron and ascorbic acid', *British Journal of Nutrition*, **34**, 1, 141–152.
50. I.I. Brekhman ,P.S. Zorikov and V.N. Zharsky (1973), 'A method of producing refined sugar'. Author's certificate (patent) No. 495355, with priority from 7 July (R).
51. Ye.V. Volf and O.F. Maleyeva (1969), *World Resources of Useful Plants*, 'Nauka', Leningrad (R); A.A. Pristupa (1973), *Basic Raw-Material Plants and their Use*, 'Nauka', Leningrad (R); and W. Karrer (1958), *The Constitution and Occurrence of Organic Vegetable Matter*, Birkhäuser Verlag, Basel and Stuttgart (G).
52. The English word 'stamina' — meaning constitutional strength, endurance, perseverance, and resistance — derives from the same Latin word that forms the basis of thread or tissue [Specifically, the threads spun by the Fates determining length of life — Translator].
53. I.I. Brekhman (1957), *Ginseng*, Gosudarstvennoye izdatelstvo meditsinskoy literatury, Leningrad (R); I.I. Brekhman (1968), *Eleutherococcus*, 'Nauka', Moscow (R); I.I. Brekhman, Yu.I. Dobryakov, and A.I. Taneyeva (1968), *New Facts about the Pharmacology of Non-Ossified Deer Antlers*, Vladivostok (R); and I.I. Brekhman, Yu.I. Dobryakov, A.M. Yudin and I.F. Nesterenko (1978), 'The pharmacological characteristics of rantarin', in *The Biological Resources of East and South-east Asia and their Utilization*, Vladivostok, 90–93 (R).
54. I.I. Brekhman, V.A. Gonenko and E.Ya. Kostetsky (1971), 'The antiradiomimetic action of certain substances extracted from marine invertebrates', *Zhurnal evolyutsionnoy biokhimii i fiziologii*, **7**, 3rd series, 456–460 (R); and I.I. Brekhman, V.G. Golotin and V.A. Gonenko (1977), 'A comparative study of the antihemolytic activity of extracts and individual substances from marine invertebrates', *Comparative Biochemistry and Physiology*, **58A**, 115–117.
55. A.S. Saratikov (1973), *The golden roots (Rhodiola roses)*, Tomsk (R).
56. Our method involving swimming, and the first findings following its use, were published in 1951 (I.I. Brekhman (1951), 'A comparative assessment of the stimulant effect of different samples and preparations from ginseng root', in *Material on the Study of Stimulant and Tonic Medicines from Ginseng and Schizandra Root*, 1st series, 59–65, Vladivostok (R).

57. The instrument is an enclosed vertical plexiglass chamber, $7 \times 7 \times 25$ cm, through which a rope (an 'endless rope') moves downwards. It is set into movement by a system of pulleys connected to an electric motor through a reduction gear. The rope moves at about 6 m/min. The floor of the chamber consists of metal blades (or wires), incorporated in the mains alternating current supply (20–25 volts). Beneath it is a second floor with vertically positioned tapering metal rods which regularly, every second, and automatically are raised and move 8–10 mm over the wire floor, giving a mouse a push if it manages to sit down in such a position that the current does not affect it. The approach of exhaustion is gauged by the animals jumping down onto the floor. When completely exhausted, neither an electric current nor being pushed on by the rods will drive a mouse onto the rope. The instrument consists of four compartments, enabling a preparation always to be matched simultaneously in three doses with control. In the course of several days 10–15 or more experiments are carried out with each dose of a preparation being tested, and the same number of experiments are conducted with the control. The data obtained is plotted on a system of coordinates (the vertical axis is the average increase in work continuity compared with control in percentage terms; the horizontal axis reproduces the logarithms of the doses) and the resultant three points are joined by a straight line. Having dropped a perpendicular from the point of intersection of the straight and horizontal lines, corresponding to a 33% increase in work continuity, to the horizontal axis, the logarithms of the investigated dose are found for increasing work continuity to complete exhaustion by 33%. From a logarithm one finds the dose itself, corresponding to a fixed stimulating unit of action (SUA). Then the amount of SUAs in 1 g of the tested preparation is determined. The result obtained is taken as positive if a larger dose makes a significant difference from control in work continuity expressed in minutes. An example is given in the following table of an investigation into the activity of white and brown sugar with complete data processing:

Table influence of white and brown sugar on the work continuity of mice to complete exhaustion.

Conditions of experiments	Solution concentration	Dose, g/kg	Number of animals	Average work continuity min.	P	Increased work continuity, % control	Number of SUAs in 1 g
Control	0.9	0.15 ml	16	39.0 ± 1.4		100	
(p–p NaCl)		1.0	15	39.0 ± 2.1		100	
White		1.5	16	40.0 ± 1.87		102	
(99.75% sucrose)	20	2.2	16	43.5 ± 1.95	0.057	111	
Control	0.9	0.15 ml	15	43.0 ± 1.3		100	
(p–p NaCl)		1.0	15	51.0 ± 1.3	0.001	117	27.0
Brown		1.5	15	52.0 ± 2.0	0.001	132	
(89.1% sucrose)	20	2.2	16	60.0 ± 1.5	0.001	134	

(I.I. Brekhman, M.A. Grinevich and G.I. Glazunov (1963), 'The influence of liquid ginseng extract on the 'work' continuity of white mice to total exhaustion', *Soobshcheniya Dalnevostochnogo filiala Sibirskogo otdeleniya Akademii nauk SSSR*, 19th series, Vladivostok, 135—138 (R); I.I. Brekhman (1968), *Eleutherococcus*, 'Nauka', Leningrad (R); and I.I. Brekhman, I.F. Nesterenko, E.I. Khasina, and P.S. Zorikov (1978), 'On the influence of brown cane sugar on work capacity and manifested signs of stress in animals', *Voprosy pitaniya*, 6, 69—70 (R).

58. An examination of the physico-chemical characteristics of samples of sugar from France, the USA, Sweden and Denmark yielded the following results:

| Country | Sucrose | Indicators, % | | | |
		Accompanying substances	Reducing substances	Moisture	Ash
France	98.0	2.0	0.025	0.13	0.175
USA	93.2	6.8	0.92	0.18	0.189
Sweden	96.1	3.9	0.27	0.63	0.168
Denmark	96.5	3.5	0.28	0.57	0.190
England	89.7	10.3	0.24	1.0	0.34

59. G.P. Ellis (1959), 'The Maillard reaction', in *Advances in carbohydrate chemistry*, 14, edited by L. Wolfrom, Academic Press, New York and London, 63—134. We are most indebted to Dr. N.V. Molodtsov for the division of the molasses into fractions.

60. The influence of a preliminary week's dosage of sucrose or brown sugar on the weight (mg/100 g) of certain internal organs of rats under stress (suspended by the fold in the skin of the neck for 18 hours):

| Indicators | Intact: unaffected | Stress | | |
		Physiological solution	Sucrose, 15 g/kg	Brown sugar, 15 g/kg
Thymus	241 ± 24	196 ± 15	178 ± 15	215 ± 22
Spleen	333 ± 17	251 ± 18	258 ± 17	276 ± 26
Thyroid gland	12 ± 0.8	14.2 ± 1.0	14.0 ± 1.3	15.5 ± 1.2
Adrenal glands	16 ± 1.1	21 ± 1.3	22 ± 1.5	24 ± 1.6
Liver (g/100 g)	4.2 ± 0.5	4.4 ± 0.3	4.4 ± 0.3	4.4 ± 0.4
Kidneys	829 ± 26	884 ± 25	879 ± 37	879 ± 34
Number of animals	54	64	65	63
"Stress index"	0	7	9	7

61. The influence of different kinds of molasses on the average number of stomach mucous haemorrhages during stress (rats suspended for 18 hours by the fold in the skin of the neck):

Experiment conditions	Dose, ml/100 g	Molasses		
		White	Green	Brown
Intact	—	0	0	0
Physiological solution (control)	1.2	0.8	1.7	1.9
Sucrose	1.2	0.4	1.0	2.0
Molasses	0.6	0.2	0.83	1.7
"	1.2	0.6	0.6	0.8
"	2.4	0.5	0.2	0.2

(left margin vertical label: STRESS)

62. The influence of a preliminary fortnight's dosage of white or brown sugar on the manifestation of stress reaction in rats, induced by being suspended for 24 hours:

Conditions of experiments	Blood sugar, mg %	Blood β-lipoproteins, mg %	Liver glycogen, mg/g	Blood deoxycorticosteroids, mg %
1. Norm	86 ± 5.2	136 ± 8.9	38 ± 8.6	16.7 ± 2.9
2. Control	128 ± 4.2 $P < 0.001$ 1–2	210 ± 10.6 $P < 0.001$ 1–2	12.9 ± 2.3 $P < 0.05$ 1–2	48.5 ± 3.6 $P < 0.01$ 1–2
3. White sugar, 15 g/kg	120 ± 4.9 $P < 0.001$ 1–3	198 ± 6.4 $P < 0.001$ 1–3	15.9 ± 4.2	56.2 ± 4.2 $P < 0.01$ 1–3
4. Brown sugar, 15 g/kg	90 ± 7.8 $P < 0.05$ 2–4	150 ± 10.1 $P < 0.01$ 2–4	25.8 ± 3.7 $P < 0.05$ 2–4	30.0 ± 4.8 $P < 0.05$ 2–4

(left margin vertical label: STRESS)

63. The influence of a preliminary fortnight's dosage with a mixture of six organic acids on the manifestation of stress reaction in rats, induced by being suspended for 24 hours:

Conditions of experiments	Blood sugar, mg %	Blood β-lipoproteins, mg, %	Liver glycogen mg/g	Blood ii-deoxy-corticosteroids, mg, %
1. Norm	84 ± 6.0	122 ± 10.4	39.2 ± 8.2	18.4 ± 2.1
2. Control	115 ± 4.6 $P < 0.001$ 1–2	190 ± 10.2 $P < 0.01$ 1–2	12.6 ± 4.2 $P < 0.05$ 1–2	48.2 ± 4.4 $P < 0.001$ 1–2
3. Total organic acids, 70 mg/kg	90 ± 5.1 $P < 0.05$ 2–3	136 ± 8.6 $P < 0.01$ 2–3	24.4 ± 3.2 $P < 0.05$ 2–3	28.6 ± 2.4 $P < 0.01$ 2–3

(left margin vertical label: STRESS)

64. R.L. Hays, E.W. Hahn and K.A. Kendall (1965), 'Evidence for decreased steroidogenesis in pregnant rats fed a sucrose diet', *Endocrinology*, **76**, 4, 771–772.

65. A.P. Dyban (1962), 'Histophysiological and experimental research on certain questions of pathological embryology in man', *Vestnik Akademii meditsinskikh nauk*, 11, 51—60 (R).

66. On ginseng's toxicity see: I.I. Brekhman (1957), *Ginseng*, Gosudarstvennogo izdatelstvo meditsinskoy literatury, Leningrad (R); S.K. Udalov (1963), 'A case of poisoning by a tincture of ginseng root', *Materialy k izucheniyu zhenshenya i drugikh lekarstvennukh rasteniy Dalnego Vostoka*, 5th series, Vladivostok, 167—169 (R); and R.K. Siegal (1979), 'Ginseng abuse syndrome. Problems with the panaceae', *Journal of the American Medical Association*, 241, 15, 1614—1615.

67. R.J. William, J.D. Heffley, Man-Li Yew and C.W. Bode (1973), 'The 'trophic' value of foods', *Proceedings of the National Academy of Sciences, USA*, 70, 3, 710—713.

68. In ali likelihood Yudkin has in mind L.W. Daldrup's and W. Wisser's 'Influence of extra sucrose with daily food on the life-span of Wistar albino rats', *Nature (London)*, 222, 5198, 1050—1052 (1969).

69. Based on C.A. Winter's and S. Flataker's method, modified by K.A. Meshcherskaya and G.M. Goncharova. (K.A. Meshcherskaya and G.M. Goncharova (1969), 'Some changes in Winter's and Flataker's method of the primary selection of neurotropic medicines', in *Materials of the conference for the pharmacology of central cholinomimetics and other neurotropic medicines*, Leningrad, 266—268) (R).

70. Based on the method of W.N. Boyer, N.A. Cross and C. Anderson (1974), 'Quality reward preference in the rat', *Bulletin of the Psychonomic Society*, 3, 5, 332—334.

71. I.I. Brekhman, I.F. Nesterenko, E.I. Khasina and P.S. Zorikov (1978), 'The influence of brown cane sugar on work capacity and the manifestation of signs of stress in animals', *Voprosy pitaniya*, 6, 69—70 (R); and I.F. Nesterenko and E.I. Khasina (1977), 'Brown Sugar's antistress action', in the collection *Theses of reports of the Second All-Union Conference for man's adaptation to different geographical, climatic and production conditions*, 2, Novosibirsk, 25—26 (R).

72. S.U. Cohen and A. Tutelbaum (1964), 'Effect of dietary sucrose and starch on oral glucose tolerance and insulin-like activity', *American Journal of Physiology*, 206, 1, 105—108 and A.M. Cohen, J.C. Michelson, and L. Larno (1972), 'Retinopathie in rats with distributed carbohydrate metabolism following a high sucrose diet', *American Journal of Opthalmology*, 73, 6, 813—869.

73. K. Brunk (1967), 'Spontaneous diabetes mellitus in dogs', *Berliner und Münchener therapeutische Wochenschrift*, 80, 22, 433—436 (G); and W. Gepts and D. Toussaint (1967), 'Spontaneous diabetes in dogs and cats. A pathological study', *Diabetologica*, 3, 2, 249—265.

74. V.F. Markelova and B.G. Lyapkov (1971), 'The dependence of the metabolic processes on the combination of qualitatively different carbohydrates and fats in diet', *Voprosy pitaniya*, **6**, 3—6 (R); V.F. Markelova and Yu.M. Zalesskaya (1974), 'Particular aspects of sucrose's influence on lipid metabolism based on the level of fats in diet', *Byulleten eksperimentalnoy biologii i meditsini*, **5**, 41—44 (R); the same authors (1974), 'Special features of lipid synthesis in conditions of prolonged imbalance in the food intake of rats', *Voprosy meditsinskoy khimii*, **2**, 198—203 (R); and V.F. Markelova and E.F. Istratenkova (1977), 'The question of sucrose's influence on the intensity of changes in lipid metabolism in protein dietary deficiency', *Voprosy pitaniya*, **2**, 29—33 (R).

75. A.E. Bender and P. Thalan (1970), 'Some metabolic effects of dietary sucrose', *Nutrition and Metabolism*, **1**, 22—39; and P. Nestel, K. Carrol, and I.V. Havenstin (1970), 'Plasma triglyceride response to carbohydrates, fats and caloric intake', *Metabolism*, **19**, 1, 1—18.

76. Y. Groen (1973), 'Why bread in the diet lowers serum cholesterol?', *Proceedings of the Nutrition Society*, **32**, 3, 159—167; D. Kritchevsky, S.A. Teppe and Y.K. Story (1975), 'Nonnutritive fiber and lipid metabolism', *Journal of Food Science*, **40**, 1, 8—11; and G.S. Ranhorte (1973), 'Effect of cellulose and wheat mill-fractions on plasma and liver cholesterol fed rats, *Cereal Chemistry*, **58**, 3, 588—603.

77. The influence of different amounts of white and brown sugar on certain indicators of the carbohydrate metabolism of rats (in an experiment lasting 90 days):

Sugar dose, g/kg	Experimental conditions	Blood sugar, mg %	Glycogen, mg %	
			Liver	Muscle
—	Control	119 ± 3.5	3680 ± 340	275 ± 18
2	White sugar	126 ± 8.5	4420 ± 400	359 ± 20
	Brown sugar	124 ± 6.5	3640 ± 78	310 ± 16 P = 0.073
15	White sugar	130 ± 4.4	4400 ± 89	482 ± 30
	Brown sugar	117 ± 6.8	3370 ± 85 P < 0.001	394 ± 28 P < 0.001
—	Control	89 ± 3.4	3130 ± 63	183 ± 16
50	White sugar	110 ± 6.4	3130 ± 69	265 ± 40
	Brown sugar	93 ± 2.0 P = 0.022	3235 ± 126	515 ± 23

78. The influence of different amounts of white and brown sugar on certain indicators of lipid metabolism in an experiment lasting 90 days.

Sugar dose, g/kg	Experiment conditions	Blood serum		Liver	
		Cholesterol, mg %	β-lipoproteins, mg %	Cholesterol, mg %	Total fat, mg %
–	Control	100 ± 1	109 ± 4	219 ± 15	4950 ± 256
2	White sugar	160 ± 11	145 ± 8	376 ± 20	5930 ± 114
	Brown sugar	108 ± 5	112 ± 7	322 ± 10	5630 ± 91
		P = 0.003	P = 0.011		
15	White sugar	175 ± 7	208 ± 11	404 ± 6	7170 ± 224
	Brown sugar	112 ± 5	161 ± 4	344 ± 4	5980 ± 182
		P < 0.001	P = 0.005	P < 0.001	
–	Control	75 ± 3	112 ± 6	240 ± 9	7000 ± 500
50	White sugar	110 ± 3	184 ± 15	230 ± 8	6900 ± 600
	Brown sugar	77 ± 4	112 ± 9	260 ± 9	8600 ± 900
		P < 0.001	P < 0.001		

79. G.N. Jenkins (1966), 'The refinement of foods in relation to dental caries', *Advances of Oral Biology*, **2**, 67–100; R.L. Hartles (1967), 'Carbohydrate consumption and dental caries', *American Journal of Clinical Nutrition*, **20**, 2, 152–156; G. Davies (1968), 'Dietary control of dental caries', *Alabama Journal of Medical Sciences*, **5**, 3, 284–287; L.J. Baume (1969), 'Caries prevalence and caries intensity among 12,344 schoolchildren of French Polynesia', *Archives of Oral Biology*, **14**, 2, 181–205; A.I. Marchenko and A.G. Krivoruk (1970), 'An experimental model of dental caries in golden hamsters'. In the collection: *Problemy terapevticheskoy stomatologii*, 5th series, 3–6 (R); A. Bucko (1977), 'The influence of nutrition on the evolution of teeth and dental caries', *Médicine et nutrition*, **13**, 4, 255–260 (F); and A. Scheinin and K.K. Mäkinen (1977), 'The influence of the consumption of certain sugars on caries formation in man', *Czas. stomatol.*, **30**, 6, 481–489 (Polish).

80. G.D. Campbell (1975), 'Efficiency of the human mouth as an extractor of sucrose from cane — A biological study', *Proceedings of the Annual Congress of the South African Sugar Technological Association*, **49**, 41–42; and G.D. Campbell (1976), 'A possible health factor in raw can juice and molasses', *The South African Journal*, **60**, 8, 405–408.

81. W.M. Edgar, A.J. Rugg-Gunn, G.N. Jenkins and D.–A.M. Geddes (1978), 'Photographic and direct visual recording of experimental caries-like changes in human dental enamel', *Archives of Oral Biology*, **23**, 8, 667–673.

82. W.M. Edgar, D.–A.M. Geddes, G.N. Jenkins, A.J. Rugg-Gunn and R. Howell (1978), 'Effects of calcium glycerophosphate and sodium fluoride on the induction *in vivo* of caries-like changes in human dental enamel', *Archives of Oral Biology*, **23**, 8, 655–661.

83. G.N. Jenkins (1968), 'Diet and caries: protective factors', *Alabama Journal of Medical Sciences*, **5**, 3, 276–283; and T.H. Grenby (1975), 'The control of dental decay. A review of protective chemicals for use as food additives', *Chemistry and Industry*, **4**, 166–171.

84. T.W.B. Osborn, J.N. Noriskin and J. Staz (1937), 'A comparison of crude and
     refined sugar and cereals in their ability to produce *in vitro* decalcification of
     teeth', *Journal of Dental Research*, **16**, 165—171.

85. G.N. Jenkins and F.C. Smales (1966), 'The potential importance in caries pre-
     vention of solubility reducing and antibacterial factors in unrefined plant
     products', *Archives of Oral Biology*, **11**, 6, 599—608; A. Strålfors (1966),
     'The effect of whole and defatted cocoa, and the absence of activity in cocoa
     fat', *Archives of Oral Biology*, **11**, 2, 149—161; A. Strålfors (1967), 'Effect
     on hamster caries by purine derivatives, vanillin and some tannin-containing
     materials. Caries in relation to food consumption and animal growth', *Arch-
     ives of Oral Biology*, **12**, 3, 321—332; K.G. König, and T.H. Grenby (1965),
     'The effect of wheat grain fractions and sucrose mixtures on rat caries de-
     veloping in two strains of rats maintained on different regimes and evaluated
     by two different methods', *Archives of Oral Biology*, **10**, 1, 143—153; and
     T.H. Grenby and J.B. Hutchinson (1969), 'The effects of diets containing
     sucrose, glucose and fructose on experimental dental caries in two strains of
     rats', *Archives of Oral Biology*, **14**, 4, 373—380.

86. A. Strålfors (1966), 'Inhibition of hamster caries by substances in brown
     sugar', *Archives of Oral Biology*, **11**, 6, 617—626.

87. The nature of the complaints during the first month's adaptation to moun-
     tainous conditions:

Complaints	During the first days for all 60 under test	30 days after dosage	
		White sugar, 30 people	Brown sugar, 30 people
1	2	3	4
Headache	18/30%	5/17%	3/10%
Giddiness	11/18%	3/10%	3/10%
Dysnpnoea	37/62%	8/27%	4/13%
Tachycardia	32/53%	6/20%	4/13%
Reduced appetite	46/77%	4/13%	1/3%
Increased fatiguability	48/80%	10/33%	4/13%
Somnolence	24/40%	2/7%	—/—
Difficulty in falling asleep	20/33%	—/—	—/—
Irritability	14/23%	2/7%	1/3%
Debility	38/63%	4/13%	1/3%

88. Friedrich Engels (1931), 'The role of labour in the process of humanizing the
     ape', in *The Dialectics of Nature*, 5th edition, Gosudarstvennoye sotsialno-
     economicheskoye izdatelstvo, Moscow-Leningrad, 61—73.(R).

Index

93